GROUP COGNITIVE THERAPY FOR ADDICTIONS

Also from Bruce S. Liese and Aaron T. Beck

For more information, visit the website of the Beck Institute
for Cognitive Behavior Therapy: *www.beckinstitute.org*

FOR GENERAL READERS

The Anxiety and Worry Workbook: The Cognitive Behavioral Solution
David A. Clark and Aaron T. Beck

FOR PROFESSIONALS

Cognitive Therapy of Anxiety Disorders: Science and Practice
David A. Clark and Aaron T. Beck

Cognitive Therapy of Depression
Aaron T. Beck, A. John Rush, Brian F. Shaw, and Gary Emery

Cognitive Therapy of Personality Disorders, Second Edition
Aaron T. Beck, Arthur Freeman, Denise D. Davis, and Associates

Cognitive Therapy of Substance Abuse
*Aaron T. Beck, Fred D. Wright, Cory F. Newman,
and Bruce S. Liese*

Cognitive Therapy for Adolescents in School Settings
Torrey A. Creed, Jarrod Reisweber, and Aaron T. Beck

Cognitive Therapy with Inpatients: Developing a Cognitive Milieu
*Edited by Jesse H. Wright, Michael E. Thase,
Aaron T. Beck, and John W. Ludgate*

The Integrative Power of Cognitive Therapy
Brad A. Alford and Aaron T. Beck

Schizophrenia: Cognitive Theory, Research, and Therapy
Aaron T. Beck, Neil A. Rector, Neal Stolar, and Paul Grant

GROUP COGNITIVE THERAPY FOR ADDICTIONS

Amy Wenzel
Bruce S. Liese
Aaron T. Beck
Dara G. Friedman-Wheeler

THE GUILFORD PRESS
New York   London

© 2012 The Guilford Press
A Division of Guilford Publications, Inc.
72 Spring Street, New York, NY 10012
www.guilford.com

Printed in the United States of America

This book is printed on acid-free paper.

Last digit is print number: 9 8 7 6 5 4 3 2 1

The authors have checked with sources believed to be reliable in their efforts to
provide information that is complete and generally in accord with the standards
of practice that are accepted at the time of publication. However, in view of the
possibility of human error or changes in behavioral, mental health, or medical
sciences, neither the authors, nor the editor and publisher, nor any other party who
has been involved in the preparation or publication of this work warrants that the
information contained herein is in every respect accurate or complete, and they are
not responsible for any errors or omissions or the results obtained from the use of
such information. Readers are encouraged to confirm the information contained in
this book with other sources.

Library of Congress Cataloging-in-Publication Data is available from the publisher.

ISBN 978-1-4625-0549-4

About the Authors

Amy Wenzel, PhD, is a Clinical Associate in Psychiatry at the University of Pennsylvania School of Medicine and has held faculty positions at the University of North Dakota and the American College of Norway. She is the recipient of awards from the National Alliance for Research on Schizophrenia and Depression, the American Foundation for Suicide Prevention, and the National Institutes of Health. In addition to her scholarly work, Dr. Wenzel provides training and consultation in cognitive behavioral therapy to clinicians across the United States, and she lectures nationally on cognitive behavioral approaches to the understanding and treatment of psychiatric disorders. She is on the scientific advisory board of the American Foundation for Suicide Prevention and has held leadership positions with the Association for Behavioral and Cognitive Therapies. Dr. Wenzel is the author or editor of nine books, many of which are focused on cognitive theory and therapy, and she has published approximately 100 scholarly articles and chapters on cognitive therapy, cognitive processing, and psychopathology.

Bruce S. Liese, PhD, ABPP, is Professor of Family Medicine at the University of Kansas Medical Center, where he has taught and practiced psychology for almost three decades. A Fellow of the American Psychological Association (Division 50—Society of Addiction Psychology) and a Diplomate of the American Board of Professional Psychologists, specializing in Family Psychology, Dr. Liese has done extensive research, teaching, and practice in the field of addictive behaviors. He served as editor of *The Addictions Newsletter* for the Society of Addiction Psychology from 1993 to 2003, and in 2003 received the Society's Presidential Citation for Distinguished

Service. One of the most fulfilling experiences of Dr. Liese's career was collaborating with Aaron T. Beck, Fred D. Wright, and Cory F. Newman on their seminal text, *Cognitive Therapy of Substance Abuse* (1993). It was this work that ultimately led to the current volume on group cognitive therapy for addictions.

Aaron T. Beck, MD, is University Professor Emeritus of Psychiatry, School of Medicine, University of Pennsylvania, and the founder of cognitive therapy. Dr. Beck is the recipient of numerous awards, including the Albert Lasker Clinical Medical Research Award, the American Psychological Association Lifetime Achievement Award, the American Psychiatric Association Distinguished Service Award, the Robert J. and Claire Pasarow Foundation Award for Research in Neuropsychiatry, and the Institute of Medicine's Sarnat International Prize in Mental Health and Gustav O. Lienhard Award. He is President of the Beck Institute for Cognitive Behavior Therapy and Honorary President of the Academy of Cognitive Therapy.

Dara G. Friedman-Wheeler, PhD, is Assistant Professor of Psychology at Goucher College in Baltimore, Maryland, and a licensed psychologist. Dr. Friedman-Wheeler has received several awards from the National Institutes of Health. Her research interests are in the areas of coping, affect regulation, outcome expectancies, mood disorders, and health behaviors/outcomes. Her current research includes projects in mood-regulation expectancies for specific coping strategies and reminiscence as a therapeutic intervention. She has worked on projects in the areas of cigarette smoking and other addictions, pain, chronic multisymptom illnesses, mood disorders, and suicide, and has coauthored journal articles on cigarette smoking, mood disorders, outcome expectancies, and coping.

Preface

The treatment described in this volume has benefited from two decades of development and refinement. Led by the efforts of Bruce Liese, it has emerged from applying the principles and strategies described in the seminal book *Cognitive Therapy of Substance Abuse* (A. T. Beck, Wright, Newman, & Liese, 1993) to a group format. This treatment harnesses the power of group dynamics (e.g., group cohesiveness) while simultaneously promoting tangible strategies for achieving lasting cognitive and behavioral change. In addition, it is grounded in a comprehensive psychological theory of addiction, which itself was informed by evidence-based constructs that have been identified in the empirical literature. Perhaps the most appealing characteristic of this treatment is its flexibility: it can be implemented in a wide range of treatment settings and is appropriate for patients who struggle with a wide array of addictive behaviors.

Readers might ask why the field needs another psychotherapy for addiction, let alone another *cognitive behavioral* treatment. Indeed, there exist a number of cognitive behaviorally based treatment protocols that are efficacious in treating particular addictions (e.g., Marlatt & Donovan, 2005; Monti, Kadden, Rohsenow, Cooney, & Abrams, 2002; L. C. Sobell & Sobell, 2011). We do not approach this quandary from an "either–or" standpoint, such that we advocate for patients with addictions to receive one but not the other treatments. In fact, our treatment was heavily influenced by the theory and strategy associated with these protocols. As the reader sees in Chapter 1, we know that people who struggle with addictions need treatment, and they often do not get it, or they do not get enough of it. The treatment we describe in this volume derives from clinical research and can be used in conjunction with any legitimate addiction treatment approach. It provides yet another option for patients who often have difficulty committing to treatment and are ambivalent about change. Moreover, it provides a treatment option for patients who struggle with addictions that have received less attention in the empirical literature, such as those related to pornography use, Internet use, and overeating.

As we describe in greater detail in Chapter 1, there are a number of features of this treatment that will appeal to clinicians and patients alike. This treatment is an open group, meaning that it runs continuously, and it was designed to target a wide array of addictive behavior. What this means is that patients (and clinicians) do not have to wait an inordinate amount of time to assemble enough patients with a particular type of addiction. Assuming there is space in the group, patients can be enrolled as indicated. This open format increases the likelihood that a quorum of patients will attend each week, and it enhances the generalization of cognitive behavioral principles and skills, as patients see that similar psychological processes are at work across addictive disorders. In addition, there is no prescribed curriculum that must be covered at any one time, other than brief psychoeducation about the cognitive model toward the beginning of each session. This characteristic of the treatment ensures that facilitators can respond to the needs of the group at any time, and that each session stands alone—meaning that even if a person attends only one group, he or she will be able to take away a meaningful framework to understand and address his or her addiction. These features of the group make it more likely to fit "real-life" settings where lack of attendance and dropout are common.

We wrote this book for the broad array of practitioners who work with patients with addictions—certified drug and alcohol counselors, clinical social workers, psychologists, psychiatric nurses, psychiatrists, and so on. One potentially controversial aspect of the treatment is that it is grounded in the philosophy of harm reduction, which recognizes that some patients prefer controlled engagement in an addictive behavior to abstinence. Although we believe harm reduction is consistent with many general principles of cognitive therapy (e.g., collaboration, respect for individual differences), this treatment can certainly be implemented in programs that advocate for abstinence. The cognitive and behavioral strategies described in this volume apply equally to patients who are working toward controlled engagement in their addictive behavior and patients who are committed to abstinence. The keys in implementing the treatment from either philosophical stance are to ensure that patients are in agreement with the goals, buy into the model, and believe their viewpoints and experiences are respected.

This volume is organized in three parts. In Part I, readers receive an orientation to the problem and the general treatment approach. They learn about theory that underlies the cognitive behavioral treatment of addiction as well as theory that pertains to group dynamics. In Part II, readers learn about the main components of the treatment. After reading this part, readers will have been exposed to an array of cognitive and behavioral strategies that they can use with their patients in the group setting. In Part III, readers have an opportunity to pull the information together and contemplate the full array of treatment targets and corresponding strategies that can be implemented over the life of the treatment. Moreover, readers are introduced to other issues that are critical to consider when conducting group psychotherapy, such as dealing with difficult patients and ensuring that there is a defined end of treatment for individual group members. We encourage readers to read the full manual before conducting a group and to consult the manual as needed as specific issues arise. We also strongly encourage readers to consult the other treatment manuals that are highlighted in this volume. There is a rich array of cognitive and behavioral strategies that experts have spent decades developing, testing, and refining. We could not do all of these strategies justice in this volume, but they can all be integrated into the treatment approach if they are indicated from the conceptualization of patients' clinical presentations.

Before closing, we would like to extend our heartfelt gratitude to the staff at Guilford Publications for believing in this treatment and ensuring that this volume reached publication. Jim Nageotte worked for several years with us to make this volume become a reality. His patience is unmatched. We also appreciate the support and effort from Seymour Weingarten and Jane Keislar. Without the three of you, this project would not have come to fruition.

Contents

PART I   BACKGROUND

INTRODUCTION TO PART I

Addiction is a major public health problem, as it is often associated
with substantial financial cost, emotional distress, legal problems,
health concerns, and/or interpersonal strife. There are a number of
treatment options available to people who struggle with addictions,
ranging from peer-led groups like Alcoholics Anonymous to profes-
sionally developed inpatient treatment programs. Researchers have
received millions of dollars of government funding to understand
the nature of addiction, its course, the mechanisms that maintain
addictive behavior, and effective treatments. Although scholars
and lay people alike have significantly increased their knowledge
about addiction over the past several decades, addiction continues
to affect a substantial minority of the population. Moreover, treatments for addiction have been shown to be more effective than no
treatment, but there are high relapse rates associated with even the
most carefully developed and evaluated treatments. Thus, there
continues to be a pressing need to develop and refine additional
treatments options for addictive behavior.

Part I provides background information that will facilitate
the implementation of one specific treatment for addiction—the

1

cognitive therapy addictions group (CTAG). In Chapter 1, readers learn about the scope of the problem, including statistics that illustrate the widespread engagement in addictive behavior and the number of people who struggle with addictive disorders. In addition, readers learn about one particular modality of treatment whose efficacy has been supported in the empirical literature—cognitive therapy. This chapter explains the manner in which the CTAG has built upon the principles of cognitive therapy and has been adapted on the basis of contemporary thinking about addiction. In Chapter 2, readers learn about a psychological model of addiction that was developed from a previous cognitive model of addiction and that was modified on the basis of other important psychological factors that have been identified in the empirical literature. In Chapter 3, readers learn about factors inherent to any group treatment approach, as well as ways to conceptualize patients' readiness for change. In Chapter 4, readers become oriented to the main components for the CTAG, each of which is described in greater length in chapters in Part II. Finally, in Chapter 5, readers are introduced to the concept of cognitive case conceptualization and learn how to apply the psychological model of addiction to their patients and the group as a whole. After reading Part I readers come away with an understanding of the psychological factors that contribute to the development and maintenance of addiction, ways to address these factors by harnessing the power of group therapy, and ways to apply these concepts to any one patient.

CHAPTER 1 | Scope of the Problem

Addiction is a major public health problem that is associated with substantial adverse consequences for families, communities, health care access and provision, and addicted individuals themselves. According to the American Society of Addiction Medicine (ASAM), *addiction* is defined as "a primary, chronic disease of brain reward, motivation, memory, and related circuitry" and "is characterized by inability to consistently abstain, impairment in behavioral control, craving, diminished recognition of significant problems with one's behaviors and interpersonal relationships, and a dysfunctional emotional response" (n.d.).

There are many notable features of this definition. First, by referring to an addiction as a "chronic disease," this definition points to the lifelong struggle that many individuals with addictions endure. Second, by referring to "brain reward, motivation, memory, and related circuitry," this definition implies that addiction has a significant neurobiological component. Third, by referring to an array of consequences of addiction, this definition acknowledges that addiction is associated with significant individual and relational impairment and distress.

Notice, however, that this definition does not reference any particular type of addictive behavior. This reflects contemporary conceptualizations of addiction, which suggest that addictive behavior characterizes much more than the misuse of alcohol and drugs (Freimuth, 2005; J. E. Grant, Brewer, & Potenza, 2006). The current diagnostic manual, the *Diagnostic and Statistical Manual of Mental Disorders* (DSM-IV-TR; American Psychiatric Association, 2000), includes misuse of alcohol, illicit drugs, prescription drugs, nicotine, and caffeine in the broad category of substance-related disorders.

The DSM-IV-TR recognizes two kinds of substance misuse: (1) abuse and (2) dependence. *Abuse* is characterized by a problematic pattern of substance use that is associated with life interference within a 12-month period. Examples of life interference include a failure to perform expected duties at work or at home, using the substance in potentially dangerous situations (e.g., drinking and driving), legal consequences of substance use, and interpersonal strife resulting from the substance use. *Dependence* is also characterized by a problematic pattern of substance use that is associated with life interference within a 12-month period. However, in most instances, the consequences of dependence are even more severe and persistent than those associated with abuse. These consequences can include tolerance, withdrawal, unsuccessful attempts at decreasing use, and the devotion of a significant amount of time to substance use at the expense of other important occupational, social, or recreational activities. Many experts refer to *substance use disorders* as those that involve either the abuse or dependence of alcohol or drugs.

These diagnostic criteria are likely to change with the publication of DSM-5 (American Psychiatric Association, 2010). However, a new set of criteria will not change the fact that a significant number of people will be addicted to alcohol, drugs, and other behaviors, such as gambling and compulsive sexual behavior, and that these people are in serious need of effective treatment. Research sponsored by the Substance Abuse and Mental Health Services Administration (SAMHSA; 2011) indicates that rates of alcohol and drug dependence have been relatively stable across the first decade of the 21st century. This finding suggests that treatment programs and public health initiatives have not been successful in decreasing the rates of the addictions that have received the most attention in clinical settings and in the research literature.

This volume describes a treatment for addictions that recognizes many of the key components of addictive behavior described thus far. The cognitive therapy addictions group (CTAG) is a group treatment approach that has its basis in cognitive behavioral therapy (CBT), an active, semi-structured approach to treatment that focuses on the establishment of healthy patterns of thinking and behavior. CTAGs welcome members who are at any point in their journey of recovering from addiction, recognizing that addiction is a chronic problem and that people who have struggled with addiction are prone to relapse. The model underlying the CTAG recognizes that there are biological substrates that increase some people's vulnerability to addiction and that biological changes result from chronic engagement in addictive behavior. CTAGs directly address the myriad adverse consequences of addictive behavior to the individual and family and provide group members with tangible cognitive and behavioral strategies to manage these consequences. Finally, CTAGs are open to people with a wide range of addictions—not only alcohol and drug use—in light of the fact that many of the same cognitive and behavioral processes are at work in addiction despite the diversity of addictive behaviors (cf. Flores, 2007).

PREVALENCE AND COST OF ADDICTIONS

It is no secret that addictions cause great disturbance in today's society. We frequently watch the evening news, read the newspaper, or peruse an Internet news site and hear of tragedies caused by people who drive while intoxicated, or of the staggering costs to society caused by alcohol and drug abuse, or of alarming new trends in Internet use or pornography viewing. In this section, we provide information on the prevalence and consequences of many addictive behaviors so that readers can understand the grave need for effective treatments and provide psychoeducation to their patients and their patients' families.

Alcohol, Drug, and Tobacco Misuse

By far, the most research and clinical attention has been devoted to alcohol, drug, and tobacco misuse, as these addictions have been recognized by health professionals and researchers alike as significant public health problems for many years. Part of the reason why alcohol, drug, and tobacco misuse is such a problem is that these behaviors are commonly accepted in today's society. Results from the 2010 National Survey on Drug Use and Health (SAMHSA, 2011) revealed that heavy drinking, defined as binge drinking on at least 5 days of the past 30 days, was reported by 6.7%, or 16.9 million people in the United States ages 12 or older. Illicit drug use, consisting of the use of drugs such as marijuana, hashish, cocaine (including crack), heroin, hallucinogens, inhalants, and prescription drugs for nonmedical reasons, has risen to its highest level in 8 years. Specifically, 22.6 million people, or 8.9% of the U.S. population ages 12 or older, said they had used illicit drugs in the month prior to the survey. Tobacco use was reported by 69.9 million Americans ages 12 or older, or 27.4% of the population in that age range. In fact, according to a survey by the World Health Organization (WHO), the United States led the 16 other nations surveyed, spanning North and South America, Europe, Asia, Africa, and Australia, in lifetime use of cocaine, cannabis, and tobacco (Degenhardt et al., 2008). Clearly, use of alcohol, drugs, and tobacco is a part of American culture for a substantial minority of people.

The number of Americans who meet criteria for a substance use disorder is equally as alarming. According to results from the National Epidemiologic Survey on Alcohol and Related Conditions (Stinson et al., 2005), in

2001–2002, 7.4% of adults in the United States ages 18 or older met criteria for a current alcohol use disorder (i.e., abuse or dependence), 0.9% for a current drug use disorder, and 1.1% for a current co-occurring alcohol and drug use disorder. In other words, over 9% of American adults met diagnostic criteria for a current alcohol or drug use disorder. These rates more than triple when one considers the percentage of the population who has met criteria for one of these conditions at some point in their lives (Hasin, Stinson, Ogburn, & Grant, 2007). SAMHSA's National Survey on Drug Use and Health (2011) includes individuals ages 12 and older, and results indicate that 8.7% of American adolescents and adults meet criteria for a substance use disorder. Similarly, epidemiological research suggests that about 25% of Americans have been dependent on nicotine at some point in their lives (Breslau, Johnson, Hiripi, & Kessler, 2001; Hughes, Helzer, & Lindberg, 2006), with 15% meeting criteria for current nicotine dependence (Hughes et al., 2006).

The consequences of substance use disorders are staggering. According to the WHO, alcohol abuse is the third leading risk factor for early death and disabilities around the world. In 2004, an estimated 2.5 million people died of alcohol-related causes, including 320,000 people between ages 15 and 29 (WHO, 2010). Tobacco use is responsible for 1 in 10 adult deaths, killing more than 5 million people per year worldwide. In fact, there are approximately 1 billion smokers across the globe, and more than half of them will die prematurely of tobacco-related causes (WHO, 2011). In the United States, drug-related deaths have increased from 6.8 deaths per 100,000 in 1999 to 12.6 deaths per 100,000 in 2007. These numbers highlight a pressing need to continue developing effective prevention and intervention strategies in order to save lives.

Substance use disorders can cause health problems on multiple levels. Health problems might arise from the physiological effects of the substance (e.g., alcohol cirrhosis), from the effects of the practice of using the substance (e.g., nonsterile injections), from the behaviors in which people engage while under the influence (e.g., drinking and driving), from the consequences of the lifestyle associated with heavy substance use, or from the neglect of existing health problems (Des Jarlais, 1995; Islam, Day, & Conigrave, 2010). Despite their need for health care interventions, substance users often do not have access to health care or choose not to use it, resulting in a precarious situation in which they ultimately present for emergency treatment with acute conditions, which is of great cost to the health care system (Islam et al., 2010). In 2008, there were approximately 2 million visits to the emergency rooms in American hospitals for drug abuse/misuse—about half of those involved the use of illicit drugs, and the other half involved the nonmedical use of pharmaceuticals (SAMHSA,

2010). Moreover, substance use disorders often co-occur with psychiatric disorders, such as depression and anxiety (e.g., Hasin et al., 2007), which means that there is the potential for mental health to be affected just as much as physical health.

The resulting economic cost of substance use disorders illustrates just how great a toll on society these addictions are taking. In 2002, the economic cost of drug abuse in the United States was estimated at $180.9 billion (Office of National Drug Control Policy, 2004), which includes the resources needed to address health and crime consequences and the loss of productivity due to disability, premature death, and inability to work. In addition, it has been estimated that cigarette smoking was associated with $193 billion in health-related costs each year from 2000 to 2004, including lost productivity and direct medical costs (Centers for Disease Control and Prevention, 2008). These numbers indicate that substance use disorders affect all of us, even if we do not know a single individual who is struggling with the effects of a substance use disorder. Moreover, these numbers say nothing about the distress that substance use disorders cause to marriages, families, and other close relationships (Friedmann, Hendrickson, Gerstein, & Zhang, 2004).

Other Addictions

Only now are researchers beginning to study the prevalence and consequences of non-substance-related addictions, including (but not limited to) those in the realms of gambling, Internet, sex, and overeating (cf. J. E. Grant et al., 2006). There are no large national and international epidemiological studies, save for those that have assessed pathological gambling, that can provide the type of definitive information about these addictions that we presented in the previous section on alcohol, drug, and tobacco misuse. Nevertheless, we are starting to see that nonsubstance use addictions can be just as debilitating as substance use disorders, and in the remainder of this section, we cite the available research that is beginning to identify the prevalence and consequences of these other addictions.

Although gambling addiction has received significant attention from the research literature in the past two decades, the need to address this addictive behavior has been known at least since the late 1950s, when the first Gamblers Anonymous meeting was held (Gamblers Anonymous International Service Office, n.d.). Gambling is another potentially addictive behavior that is commonly accepted in American society. Epidemiological research indicates that over 75% of Americans report that they have gambled at least once in their lives, that over 50% of Americans report that they have gambled more than 10 times, that over 25% of Americans report that they have gambled over 100 times, and that over 10% of Americans report that they have gambled over 1,000 times (Kessler et al., 2008). The lifetime prevalence of pathological gambling, defined in a similar manner as DSM-IV-TR substance abuse and dependence, ranges from 0.6% (Kessler et al., 2008) to 1.6% (Shaffer, Hall, & Vander Bilt, 1999), although results from smaller studies raise the possibility that, in some areas of the world, the prevalence is up to 7% (Ladouceur & Walker, 1996). Pathological gambling is associated with many financial, relational, and legal consequences, including high rates of bankruptcy, divorce, and incarceration (J. E. Grant & Potenza, 2007). Like the other addictive behaviors, it is associated with high rates of comorbidity with psychiatric disorders (J. E. Grant & Potenza, 2007), which raises the possibility that gambling addiction puts people at risk for adverse mental health consequences.

In contrast to gambling, the Internet is a relatively recent phenomenon that has assumed an increasing amount of importance over the past 20 years. Although the Internet is a crucial tool for obtaining necessary information to conduct research in our professional and personal lives, it also offers a number of social and recreational outlets (e.g., gaming, social chat rooms, dating sites) that have the potential to consume a great deal of time. Up to 6% of the population reports an Internet addiction (Young, 2007). Internet addiction might not necessarily be associated with the health and mortality consequences that are associated with substance use disorders. However, research shows that it is strongly associated with social isolation and marital discord, as Internet relationships can replace "real-life" intimacy with other partners, and many people with an Internet addiction hide their behavior and lie to others about it (Brenner, 1997; Morahan-Martin & Schumacher, 1999; Young, 1998). Moreover, research shows that Internet addiction is similar to substance use disorders in that it is often used as a tool to escape life problems (Young, 2007).

Of course, a large subset of problem online behavior is Internet sex addiction, which includes visiting adult websites to view pornographic material and participating in adult chat rooms, among other activities (Young, 2008). Sex addiction (sometimes referred to as hypersexuality) that occurs primarily online, however, may represent only about one-quarter of all compulsive sexual behavior (Cooper, Delmonico, & Burg, 2000). Other manifestations of hypersexuality include compulsive masturbation, promiscuity, excessive viewing of pornographic magazines and movies, frequent attendance at strip clubs, and telephone sex (Kafka, 2007). Although it has been difficult to measure the prevalence of sex addictions, it is clear that pornography is an enormous industry in the United States (Weinberg, Williams, Kleiner, & Irizarry, 2010). In addition, compulsive sexual behavior is associated with significant relationship distress, although relationship problems are often perceived as more distressing to the partner than to the addicted individual him- or herself (Cooper, Scherer, Boies, & Gordon, 1999). When hypersexual behavior extends beyond the online community, there is an increased risk of unprotected sex (Muench et al., 2007), which, in turn, is associated with the spread of sexually transmitted diseases (Kalichman, Cherry, Cain, Pope, & Kalichman, 2005) and unintended pregnancies (McBride, Reece, & Sanders, 2008).

Finally, many experts consider overeating to be an addictive behavior. Currently, people regarded as having binge eating disorder are diagnosed with eating disorder not otherwise specified. The lifetime prevalence of binge eating disorder is estimated to be 2.8% (Hudson, Hiripi, Pope, & Kessler, 2007), and one study found that 92% of a sample of patients with binge eating disorder would meet criteria for a substance use disorder if the substance in question were binge eating, with some of these patients describing themselves as "food addicts" and "compulsive overeaters" (Cassin & von Ranson, 2007). Binge eating disorder is associated with substantial health risks, although evidence is currently mixed as to whether or not these health risks are solely attributable to the increased rates of obesity found among those with binge eating disorder (Striegel-Moore & Franko, 2008). Thus, it is important to keep in mind that, although there is a strong association between binge eating disorder and obesity, they are not one and the same, and it is likely that people with binge-eating disorder form a subset of obese individuals who are characterized by a hypersensitivity to the pleasure associated with eating and a predisposition to engage in addictive behavior (Davis et al., 2009). Research also shows that individuals with binge eating disorder suffer from psychosocial consequences, including comorbid psychiatric disorders and impaired social adjustment (Wilfley, Wilson, & Agras, 2003). Overeating is an addiction with unique properties, because unlike substance use addictions, abstinence is not an option. Instead, these patients need to acquire skills to regulate their food intake (Collins, 2005).

THE NEED FOR EFFECTIVE TREATMENT

To this point in the chapter, we have illustrated that addictions affect a substantial percentage of the population and that they are associated with severe health, economic, and interpersonal consequences. There exist many treatment options for people who struggle with addictions, including inpatient treatment facilities, day treatment and partial hospitalization programs, outpatient treatment programs, and self-help groups (e.g., Alcoholics Anonymous [AA]). Unfortunately, research suggests that only a small percentage of people with these addictions get the treatment they need.

For example, in the National Survey on Drug Use and Health (SAMHSA, 2011), it was determined that only approximately 11% of those who needed treatment for alcohol or drug misuse actually received treatment in a specialty facility. In the National Epidemiologic Survey on Alcohol and Related Conditions (Stinson et al., 2005), only 6.1% with an alcohol use disorder, 15.6% with a drug use disorder, and 21.8% with a co-occurring alcohol and drug use disorder sought treatment. When people with a substance use disorder enter into treatment, between one-third and two-thirds drop out prior to treatment completion (Dutra et al., 2008; Malat et al., 2008; Tzilos, Rhodes, Ledgerwood, & Greenwald, 2009). It is likely that a combination of factors accounts for these unfortunate facts; however, these statistics also suggest that addiction treatments need to be acceptable and tolerable for the people who are encouraged to seek them.

Another factor that makes the need for effective treatment all the more pressing is that relapse is extremely common among patients who struggle with addictive disorders (Marlatt & Witkiewitz, 2005; Polivy & Herman, 2002). In fact, many experts consider relapse as something to be expected (Dunn, 2000), such that returning to old behaviors is part of the natural cycle of change (DiClemente & Prochaska, 1998). For example, in a 10-year follow-up study of people with substance use disorders, of those who had achieved remission, approximately one-third relapsed in the first year, and approximately two-thirds relapsed at some point in the follow-up period (Xie, McHugo, Fox, & Drake, 2005). Other studies have reported alcohol and drug relapse rates of up to 90% in the first year (e.g., Hunt, Barnett, & Branch, 1971). Similarly, Cohen et al. (1989) found that only 13–14% of smokers were abstinent 6–12 months after their attempt to quit, and Brown (1989) reported that only 7% of gamblers were abstinent 2 years after their attempt to quit. High relapse rates are also the norm in the treatment of overeating and obesity (Collins, 2005) and relapse is similarly a part of the typical progression of sex addiction (Young, 2008). Thus, for treatments to be effective, they must account for the very high rates of relapse in addicted populations, and clinicians who administer them must directly address this issue with patients.

COGNITIVE THERAPY OF ADDICTIVE BEHAVIOR

We propose that cognitive therapy has the potential to be an effective treatment for the wide range of addictive disorders. According to A. T. Beck, Wright, Newman, and Liese (1993), there are a number of features of cognitive therapy that make it a good match for use with this population. First, patients gain perspective that their addictive behavior is the primary pathway by which they experience pleasure and/or get relief from distress. They acquire the understanding that unhelpful beliefs fuel addictive behavior, and they begin to modify these beliefs, as well as the belief that their addiction is due to circumstances outside of their control. Developing this understanding in the context of a collaborative therapeutic relationship gives patients a sound rationale for the treatment and empowers them to make decisions on the basis of this model, which may be more attractive to some patients with addictions than treatment approaches in which they are told what to do in an authoritative manner. In addition, cognitive therapy provides specific strategies for managing cravings, which strengthens a patient's "internal controls" and has the potential to decrease the likelihood of relapse. Finally, cognitive therapy also helps patients to combat negative emotional experiences like depression, anxiety, anger, guilt, and loneliness, which can serve as triggers for relapse (cf. Monti et al., 2002).

Cognitive therapy, often referred to as cognitive behavioral therapy (CBT), for addictions has been studied extensively in the research literature. As we evaluate this research literature, we use the terms *cognitive therapy* and *CBT* interchangeably, according to the terms most often used by the investigators who conducted the research. These terms also encompass many specific protocols developed on the basis of cognitive and behavioral principles, including Marlatt and his colleagues' Relapse Prevention approach (Marlatt & Donovan, 2005; Marlatt & Witkiewitz, 2005), L. C. Sobell and Sobell's Guided Self-Change approach (2011), and Monti and his colleagues' Coping Skills Training and Cue Exposure Treatment approaches (2002). The majority of the research we review in this section pertains to CBT for alcohol and drug use disorders, but we briefly reference the efficacy of CBT approaches to the treatment of other addictive disorders.

In general, comprehensive meta-analytic studies confirm that CBT is efficacious in treating alcohol and drug use disorders, as these patients exhibit significant reductions in alcohol and drug use posttreatment, and these reductions are greater than those achieved by physician advice and psychoeducational groups (Irvin, Bowers, Dunn, & Wong, 1999; Miller et al., 1995; Miller & Wilbourne, 2002). Moreover, there is evidence that improvement from participation in CBT can be maintained at least a year after treatment has ended, and, in some cases, that patients experience further improvement (Epstein, Hawkins, Covi, Umbricht, & Preston, 2003; Carroll et al., 1994, 2000). CBT for the treatment of alcohol and drug misuse is also efficacious in reducing co-occurring emotional distress (e.g., depression, anxiety) and improving coping (Hides et al., 2010). Similarly, it has been used effectively in treating cigarette smokers who are trying to quit (e.g., Marks & Sykes, 2002) and may be particularly efficacious for smokers who are vulnerable to depression (Kapson & Haaga, 2010). Both group and individual CBT protocols have been evaluated in the empirical literature, and data suggest that both approaches are efficacious (Rotgers & Nguyen, 2006).

Despite these positive findings, it is important to acknowledge that there are other efficacious treatments for substance use disorders. In fact, many studies have reported that other treatments, such as programs that facilitate engagement in 12-step programs, motivational interviewing, supportive–expressive therapy, and interactional group therapies, are equally as efficacious in achieving a decrease in substance use (e.g., Project MATCH Research Group, 1997; Kadden, Litt, Cooney, Kabela, & Getter, 2001; Woody, Luborsky, McLellan, & O'Brien, 1990). Further complicating matters is that research on the mechanism of action in CBT suggests that improvement in CBT does not necessarily occur through the acquisition of strategies that are emphasized and practiced (Morgenstern & Longabaugh, 2000), and that patients who participate in treatments that are not focused on the acquisition of cognitive and behavioral strategies exhibit significant improvement in the use of these skills posttreatment (Litt, Kadden, Cooney, & Kabela, 2003). Experts have speculated that important factors in explaining the efficacy of treatments for substance use disorders include the administration of the treatment by clinicians who have a great deal of experience with this population (Crits-Christoph et al., 1999) and the capitalization on patients' motivation and increased self-efficacy (Litt et al., 2003).

The treatment outcome literature is much less developed for addictions other than substance use disorders. However, data from existing studies show great promise in CBT for the treatment of these addictions. For example, CBT for gambling has been modeled after CBT for substance use disorders, with the idea that people who have gambling addictions make incorrect assumptions about probability, skill, and luck, and that CBT can help them acquire skills to modify these assumptions (Shaffer & LaPlante, 2005). Controlled studies have found that CBT for gambling is associated with significant reductions in gambling behavior and a desire to gamble, as well as an increase in perceived control, relative to waiting list control conditions (e.g., Sylvain, Ladouceur, & Boisvert, 1997; Ladouceur et al., 2001). CBT has been described as the "gold standard" treatment for conditions that overlap with some of the addictions considered in this chapter, such as obesity (Collins, 2005) and illegal sexual behavior (Wheeler, George, & Stoner, 2005), as well as Internet addiction (Young, 2007).

In sum, cognitive therapy is one of many efficacious treatments for substance use disorders, and it is currently regarded as the psychotherapy of choice for non-substance use addictions. Although research conducted to date raises the possibility that it does not exert its action in the manner that is intended, the facts that (1) it significantly reduces alcohol, drug, and smoking use, relative to no treatment and nonspecific treatments; and (2) it has been shown to be efficacious hundreds of times in the general psychotherapy literature (see Butler, Chapman, Forman, & Beck, 2006) suggest that it can play a role in addressing the grave need for effective treatment of people with addictions. Because results from some studies raise the possibility that addictions treatments are most effective when they are administered by professionals who have a great deal of experience with the population, and when they capitalize on patients' motivation for change and self-efficacy, it is logical that attention to these treatment characteristics would be important to consider in cognitive therapy.

The treatment described in this volume—the CTAG—indeed embraces these features. Although CTAGs can be implemented in any treatment setting (e.g., outpatient psychiatry clinics, private practices), they were designed to be compatible with interventions offered in addiction specialty programs, where treating professionals have rich clinical experience in working with this population. In addition, CTAGs welcome members at various stages of change, which means that some members are highly motivated to reduce their addictive behavior, whereas others may be ambivalent. These individual differences are respected, and strategies to enhance motivation are integrated into the group's work. It is usually the case that some group members have attended sessions for some time, whereas other group members have attended only a few sessions. This mixture of clientele allows seasoned group members to model the effective application of cognitive and behavioral coping strategies, which in turn has the potential to increase group members' confidence that these strategies do indeed work and that they can indeed apply them to their lives.

There are four additional characteristics of CTAGs that we believe make them an especially attractive treatment option for use with patients with addictions. As we discuss in Part II, the treatment is flexible. Although facilitators adhere to a general session structure format, there is no prescribed curriculum. There is nothing that *must* be done in a group member's Session 1, Session 2, and so on. Rather, facilitators educate about and model the cognitive behavioral approach to managing addictions while simultaneously responding to the needs of group members at the time of any one session. In other words, there is a cognitive therapy framework that guides each session, but the content and work of each session is guided by the concerns of the group members and the collaborative decision making between the group members and the facilitators. This flexible structure allows for a guiding framework on which facilitators can rely in helping group members to leave with something more than they had at the beginning of the session, but also for attention to be given to issues and crises that the facilitators could not have anticipated when they prepared for the session (which frequently happens).

A second characteristic that makes the CTAG an attractive option for use with patients with addictions is that it welcomes members with any type of addiction—alcohol use, drug use, tobacco use, gambling, Internet use, sex, overeating, and so on. This heterogeneity reflects the heterogeneity of the clientele in many treatment programs, making it practical to implement the CTAG continuously in these settings, rather than requiring a lengthy wait to accumulate a number of new patients who all have the same addiction to begin a group. Moreover, this heterogeneity illustrates the commonality among patients with addictions in terms of the cognitive and behavioral factors that maintain addictive behaviors, which are the very same factors that will be the targets of treatment. As a result, group members will see that addictions affect people from many different socioeconomic and cultural backgrounds, and they will benefit from multiple points of view and wisdom that they might not have otherwise considered (Bieling, McCabe, & Antony, 2006).

A third characteristic that makes the CTAG an attractive option for use with patients with addictions is the fact that it is an open group, which means that group members are not bound to attend a specific number of sessions, that they attend or do not attend as they please, and that new members are continually being integrated into the group. This structure has the potential to be particularly relevant for addiction specialty programs, which often see a large rate of turnover and dropout (McCarty et al., 2007). Thus, new members can join the group as there is space, which increases the likelihood that patients in need will receive treatment at the time when they need it the most, as well as the likelihood that there will be a large enough quorum on any given day to conduct meaningful group psychotherapy. This structure also has the potential to be especially tolerable to patients with addictions who are still in the process of making a commitment to change and may hesitate to commit to a prescribed course of treatment.

Because the CTAG is an open group, by definition, it is also ongoing. Many experts in the field of addictions state unequivocally that longer involvement in treatment is associated with better outcome (e.g., Flores, 2007; Rotgers & Nguyen, 2006), although we recognize that many patients with addictions, particularly those with alcohol dependence, achieve significant gains in time-limited treatments with as few as four to eight sessions (Monti et al., 2001; Rohsenow et al., 2001; L. C. Sobell, Sobell, & Agrawal, 2009). It also is quite common for patients with addictions to attend treatment sporadically, "recycling" through periods of abstinence or controlled use and periods of heavy use (Norcross, Krebs, & Prochaska, 2011). An ongoing group provides these patients with the opportunity to revisit and practice the skills they had acquired in the past in order to continue to work to overcome their addiction. Of course, we recognize that time-limited groups, rather than open groups, have the potential to be most compatible with some patients' insurance plans in this age of managed care (cf. L. C. Sobell & Sobell, 2011). However, the CTAG is designed in such a way so that group members who attend only a limited number of sessions are expected to take away many tangible strategies for managing their addictive behavior and, at the same time, so that group members who are able to attend a larger number of sessions can capitalize on their time in treatment by gaining extensive practice with the strategies and developing a sense of self-efficacy as they model the application of these strategies to others in the group.

Finally, a fourth characteristic that makes the CTAG an attractive option for use with patients with addictions is the group format itself. Interactions with people who are struggling with related problems allow for the emergence of curative factors that can come only from group, rather than individual, psychotherapy (Flores, 2007; L. C. Sobell & Sobell, 2011; see Chapter 3 for more discussion of these factors). Moreover, group formats offer up to 50% greater efficiency relative to individual psychotherapy (Morrison, 2001; L. C. Sobell et al., 2009), which allows treatment facilities to serve a large number of patients.

ORIENTATION TO THIS VOLUME

The remainder of this volume describes the theoretical basis for the treatment and the treatment's components and strategies. This volume is divided into three parts. Part I provides background information that is necessary to understand the context and rationale for CTAG components. This chapter presented information on the scope of the problem—the prevalence and consequences of addictions—as well as a brief overview of research that has evaluated the efficacy and effectiveness of cognitive behavioral approaches to treating addictions. Chapter 2 describes our comprehensive cognitive model of addiction so that readers can gain an understanding of the theoretical basis of the treatment and the manner in which intervention logically follows. Chapter 3 describes theory related to the implementation of group psychotherapy and motivation for change in order to give context for the CTAG that extends beyond scholarly work on cognitive behavioral theory, which is crucial in mobilizing group process and support and in enhancing group members' commitment to treatment. Chapter 4 provides a brief overview of the CTAG. Chapter 5 describes case conceptualization, or the manner in which the theory described in Chapters 2 and 3 can be used to understand the clinical presentations of individual group members, as well as the group as a whole. Part II provides a detailed description of the CTAG session components that were introduced in Chapter 4, including introductions (Chapter 6), evaluation of thoughts and beliefs (Chapter 7), development of coping skills (Chapter 8), and homework and closure (Chapter 9). Part III includes a concluding chapter that organizes the treatment strategies according to the comprehensive cognitive model of addiction, provides suggestions for handling challenging group members from a cognitive behavioral framework, and illustrates the ending of treatment for group members who have achieved their goals.

A few notes about the terminology that we use in this volume are in order. The reader will see that we often refer to group members as "engaging in addictive behavior." Although this phrase is, admittedly, awkward, we use it in this volume to be as inclusive as possible in representing the array of addictive behaviors reported by group members (e.g., "using" applies mainly to group members who have substance use disorders and does not apply as readily to those with many non-substance use addictions). We also refer to both *patients* and *group members* throughout the volume. We generally use the term "patients" to refer to people with addictions who seek treatment in general, and the term "group members" to people with addictions who participate in the CTAG. However, the terms can be used interchangeably, as the material we describe with reference to "patients" applies to CTAG members, and we would expect that the observations we have about "group members" would apply to patients in general who might choose to participate in the CTAG. At times, we refer to a patient with an addiction as "he" or "she" but the reader can assume that the information is relevant to people of both genders. Finally, we make numerous references to "slips," "lapses," and "relapse." *Slips* and *lapses* are terms that can be used interchangeably, and they refer to a single instance in which a person engages in addictive behavior after being previously abstinent, or a single instance in which a person engages excessively in addictive behavior after a period of controlled, nonharmful use. *Relapse* refers to multiple instances in which a person engages in addictive behavior after being previously abstinent, or multiple instances in which a person engages excessively in addictive behavioral after a period of controlled, nonharmful use. Often, relapse signals a return to the previous problematic pattern of behavior (Marlatt & Witkiewitz, 2005).

Throughout the volume, we follow five group members who are at various stages of change and who struggle with different types of addictions. These "case descriptions" represent a composite of characteristics that we have seen in group members whom we have treated with the CTAG. The following is a brief biography of each of these five group members.

"Dave" is a 29-year-old single Caucasian male who joined the CTAG 6 weeks earlier for polysubstance dependence, which includes heavy use of marijuana and alcohol and occasional use of crack cocaine. He recently received his second driving-under-the-influence (DUI) arrest and spent time in jail; as a result, he was ordered to enroll in the group by his probation officer. Currently, he works at an auto parts store, although he has held a number of jobs over the past 2 years and has often been fired due to being under the influence of substances at work or missing work due to being hung over. Dave lives with his girlfriend, and the two of them have an "on again, off again" relationship characterized by arguing, blaming, and occasionally, physical violence. He often goes on binges, in which he stays with his buddies for days on end. Dave expresses ambivalence, at best, about curbing his substance use; although he sees that many of his friends are "growing up" and assuming more responsibility in life, he also views substance use as an escape from his stressful home life and as a way to relive his younger years. Most of the time, Dave is defensive about his substance use, and he is often skeptical about the topics discussed in group, claiming that they do not apply to his particular situation.

"Michael" is a 45-year-old married male of mixed African American and Korean heritage who joined the CTAG 8 months earlier for a sex addition. Michael had 10 affairs with women during the time in which he was dating the woman who later became his wife and early in his marriage. He also had many additional "inappropriate" relationships with women characterized by heavy flirting, emotional intimacy, exchange of inappropriate messages (i.e., "sexting"), and occasional kissing. Immediately prior to joining the group, his wife discovered that he had been carrying on an inappropriate relationship with a coworker despite repeated promises that he would remain faithful. Michael is an attorney at a prominent firm in town, and at times he has risked his professional reputation by viewing pornography on the Internet while at work, or by engaging in inappropriate sexual behavior with female clients. Michael has two children, ages 4 and 6, and prior to joining the group, he had often missed their evening activities in order to go to strip clubs with his male colleagues, view pornography on his computer at home, or go to happy hour with female clients or colleagues. His wife has given him an ultimatum that he must stop this behavior, or she will divorce him and seek custody of the children. Michael has been abstinent from extramarital sexual and emotionally intimate behavior with other women for the past 6 months, although he continues to feel sexual tension with female coworkers whom he finds attractive or with whom he had "flirted" in the past.

"Ellen," a 61-year-old divorced Caucasian female, joined the CTAG 6 months earlier for compulsive overeating. She currently weighs 300 pounds; she joined the group at the recommendation of her doctor, who encouraged her to lose over 100 pounds. Ellen is struggling with generalizing the cognitive and behavioral strategies learned in group to her daily life. She is unemployed and receiving disability, she lives alone, and she rarely sees her adult children. She states that she is very lonely and that she has little meaning in her life. Ellen also meets criteria for major depressive disorder, and she complains of little motivation and energy to implement a structured diet and exercise routine. She finds that she overeats in the evening, when she ruminates over the fact that she lives alone and begins to view herself as worthless. She often becomes tearful in group when she admits her lack of progress to the other members.

"Allison" is a married 50-year-old Native American female who joined the CTAG a week earlier to address her nicotine addiction. Allison has smoked since age 11, and nearly all of her family members and friends also smoke. Recently, Allison has had trouble catching her breath after excessive coughing fits, and her doctor informed her that she must give up smoking in order to prevent further deterioration of her lungs. She asked her husband and her mother-in-law (who lives with her) to give up smoking with her because she became concerned with their health, and she also believed it would be easier to give up smoking if there were no cigarettes in her household. Unfortunately, her husband and mother-in-law refused to do so, and Allison constantly feels urges to smoke when she is home. She has tried nicotine gum and the patch, but she does not believe that either method has been helpful. Allison described increasing tension with her husband and mother-in-law because of this issue.

"Brian" is a 34-year-old Caucasian male who has attended the CTAG sporadically for over 2 years to address a gambling addiction. Brian had enjoyed going to the riverboat casinos to "blow off steam" ever since he turned 21 and was legally allowed to gamble, stating that he thrived on the "high" of "winning big." At age 30, his grandmother died, and he received an inheritance. Although he and his new wife had agreed to invest the money from the inheritance into their retirement, his gambling increased substantially, with the idea that he could increase the size of their newfound sum of money if he could hit the "jackpot." Eventually, Brian lost much more than he won, and he dwindled away the inheritance. Currently, Brian is separated from his wife and is struggling to make ends meet financially. His behavioral pattern is that he goes many months without gambling, but when he comes into money, he often goes to the casino and loses it. He and his wife are currently in couple's therapy in an attempt to decide whether they can repair their relationship. Brian was raised in an upper-middle-class family where achievement and success were emphasized, which contributes to the belief that he is a "loser" because of his current situation. Like Ellen, Brian meets criteria for major depressive disorder.

SUMMARY

Addictions take an enormous toll on the people who engage in addictive behavior, their families, and society as a whole. Although much funding, time, and effort have been devoted to developing efficacious treatments for addictions, the fact remains that the majority of patients who undergo treatment for addictions will relapse. Thus, scholars and clinicians must continue to develop and refine addiction treatment approaches so that they target the core factors that maintain addictive behaviors, are tolerable to patients with addictions, and address high rates of relapse. The CTAG is an outgrowth of cognitive therapy for addictions (A. T. Beck et al., 1993) that was developed to take into account these and other factors and to be administered in a flexible manner in an array of clinical settings. Though it has not yet been evaluated in a large randomized controlled trial, we view it as an *evidence-informed treatment* because its theory, structure, and strategy are firmly grounded in findings from the empirical literature (Maude-Griffin, Hohenstein, Humfleet, Reilly, Tusel, et al., 1998). This volume describes the theoretical underpinnings of the CTAG as well as the implementation of its components.

CHAPTER 2 | Theoretical Framework

A Comprehensive Cognitive Model of Addiction

Cognitive therapy is more than a collection of techniques; it is an approach to psychotherapy that includes a comprehensive theory for understanding psychological problems, emotional distress, and self-defeating behavior. A principal assumption in cognitive therapy is that emotions and behaviors are largely influenced by thought processes, including long-standing beliefs that people have about themselves, the world, and the future, as well as thoughts, images, and ideas that arise in response to particular situations or events. In addition, cognitive theory also recognizes that emotions and behavior can feed back into a person's thoughts and beliefs. By understanding the nature of long-standing beliefs, situational cognitions, and emotional and behavioral responses, cognitive therapists can identify multiple points of intervention as they are developing a treatment plan.

In this chapter, we present our cognitive model of addiction, which captures the addiction-related cognitions that are activated in situations in which a person is contemplating engaging in addictive behavior as well as long-standing factors that make the person vulnerable to experience these addiction-related cognitions when faced with triggers. This cognitive model also accounts for emotional, physiological, and behavioral reactions to these cognitions that affect the likelihood that a person will engage in addictive behavior. Much of the model has been described in previous work on cognitive therapy for addictions (A. T. Beck et al., 1993; Liese & Franz, 1996). In addition to describing these older models, we discuss other cognitive behavioral constructs that empirical research and relevant theory have identified as important in understanding addictive behavior. We illustrate the dynamic interplay between cognition and addictive behavior and demonstrate their bidirectional relation in maintaining an addictive disorder.

We conclude the chapter by presenting a comprehensive cognitive model of addiction that (1) accounts for available theory and empirical research, and (2) provides a guide for intervention.

TWO-TIERED MODEL FOR UNDERSTANDING ADDICTIVE BEHAVIOR

At its most fundament level, we view the cognitive model of addiction as consisting of two tiers (see Figure 2.1). *Proximal situational factors* are cognitive, behavioral, emotional, and physiological variables that can explain why a person engages in addictive behavior in any one situation or circumstance. We use the term, *proximal*, because these factors are at work in the time immediately prior to, during, and immediately after an episode in which a person engages in addictive behavior. These proximal factors are usually brought on by some sort of *trigger*. There is a wide range of variables that can constitute triggers, and many triggers are idiosyncratic to any one individual (Rotgers & Nguyen, 2006). For example, triggers can be external stimuli, such as the "people, places, and things" that cue people of

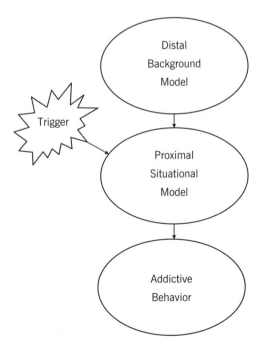

FIGURE 2.1. Two tiers for understanding addictive behavior.

previous circumstances in which they engaged in addictive behavior. Triggers can also be stressful or aversive events, such as an argument with a close other, a higher-than-average workload on the job, or a significant loss (Monti et al., 2002). However, triggers can just as easily be an internal event or stimulus, such as a particular emotional state (e.g., sadness, anxiety, anger, boredom), an unhelpful cognition (e.g., "My life isn't going anywhere"), or an uncomfortable physiological sensation (e.g., sensations that the person interprets as a craving). Moreover, triggers need not always be something negative, as they can also be positive mood states (e.g., glee) and/or an opportunity to celebrate.

The proximal situational factors that characterize any one person when he or she is triggered are just as individualized. They emerge from the person's unique profile of *distal background factors*, which are aspects of his or her personal history, genetic predisposition, personality traits, and other long-standing cognitive, emotional, behavioral, and environmental or social variables that provide a context in which the addictive behavior occurs. We use the term, *distal*, because these factors are present whether or not the person is engaging in addictive behavior and do not exert influence on a person's addiction until he or she is faced with a trigger. In other words, distal background factors can be viewed as *chronic* vulnerabilities that increase the likelihood of engaging in addictive behavior, whereas proximal situational factors can be viewed as *acute* variables that facilitate addictive behavior in response to a trigger (see Witkiewitz & Marlatt, 2004, for a similar conceptualization).

We view proximal situational factors and distal background factors as equally important to consider when conceptualizing the cognitive behavioral variables that characterize patients with addictions and in developing treatment plans with these patients. CTAGs provide a forum for patients with addictions to develop cognitive and behavioral strategies to intervene at the level of the proximal situational factors that are activated in the face of a trigger, as well as to address modifiable distal background factors that continue to make them vulnerable to slips and lapses. In the next sections, we describe specific proximal situational factors and distal background factors that cognitive theorists and empirical researchers have identified as central components of cognitive models of addiction.

Proximal Situational Factors

Basic Cognitive Model of Addiction

Figure 2.2 displays an adaptation of what has been known for the past two decades as the basic cognitive model of addiction (A. T. Beck et al., 1993; Liese & Franz, 1996). This model depicts the cognitive and behavioral

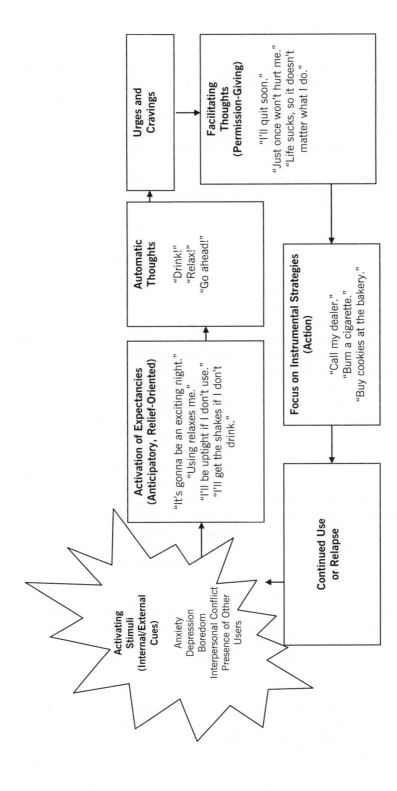

FIGURE 2.2. Basic cognitive model of addiction. Adapted from A. T. Beck et al. (1993) and Liese and Franz (1996). Copyright 1993 and 1996 by The Guilford Press. Adapted by permission.

factors at work in instances in which a person is faced with the decision of whether or not to engage in addictive behavior. The model begins with *activating stimuli*, which are the triggers that we described in Figure 2.1. As stated previously, these activating stimuli or triggers can be external or internal cues, and according to the model, they can prompt three types of unhelpful cognitions associated with addictive behavior. One type of unhelpful cognition is an addiction-related *outcome expectancy*, which is a cognition that orients the person to the anticipated effects of engaging in a particular behavior (Bandura, 1977). When a person is confronted with an activating stimulus or trigger, his or her expectancy will be focused almost exclusively on the positive effects of engaging in addictive behavior because addictions are characterized by powerful rewarding properties (Brandon, Herzog, Irvin, & Gwaltney, 2004; Jones, Corbin, & Fromme, 2001). Outcome expectancies regarding the anticipated effects of engaging in addictive behavior motivate the person to pursue those behaviors (Bandura, 1977), regardless of the degree to which the outcome expectancies are accurate (Brandon et al., 2004; Jones et al., 2001).

There are two main types of outcome expectancies reported by patients with addictions. *Anticipatory expectancies* are those that involve the anticipation of some positive addiction-related experience (e.g., "Having a few drinks will make me the life of the party," "This party will be great because it will feel good to get high"); in other words, the anticipation of positive reinforcement. According to A. T. Beck et al. (1993), common themes of anticipatory expectancies include the expectations that the addictive behavior will (1) maintain psychological and emotional balance, (2) improve social and intellectual functioning, (3) result in pleasure and excitement, (4) energize the person and provide increased power, and (5) have a soothing effect. *Relief-oriented expectancies* involve the anticipation of reduced discomfort through engaging in addictive behavior (e.g., "I can't handle stress without a drink," "I just need to get high and escape from all of this"); in other words, the anticipation of negative reinforcement. Common themes of relief-oriented expectancies include the assumptions that (1) engaging in addictive behavior will relieve boredom, tension, anxiety, and depression; and (2) cravings and associated distress will worsen unless something is done to satisfy them (A. T. Beck et al., 1993). Some patients identify more with anticipatory expectancies, and some attribute their addictive behavior primarily to relief-oriented expectancies, whereas still others describe both types of expectancies. Regardless, these expectancies fuel addictive behavior by narrowing patients' attention on the favorable outcomes of engaging in addictive behavior at the expense of the adverse consequences of engaging in addictive behavior. There is much empirical evidence that both types of outcome expectancies are associated with engagement in addictive behavior (e.g., Brandon & Baker, 1991; Pabst, Baumeister, & Kraus, 2010; Urbán & Demetrovics, 2010).

A second type of unhelpful cognition activated by the trigger is an *automatic thought*, which is a brief, spontaneous cognition that may exert a powerful influence on emotions, behaviors, and physiological processes. Automatic thoughts are abbreviated versions of anticipatory and relief-oriented expectancies in that they direct the person to engage in addictive behavior as a logical response to the expectancy. For example, people who abuse alcohol, nicotine, or other drugs might have such automatic thoughts as "Party!," "Relief!," "A beer!," or "Light up!" Automatic thoughts may also take the form of mental images, such as those shown in beer commercials (e.g., an ice-cold beer or socializing while drinking at a party). Regardless of their form, the activation of automatic thoughts brings the person one step closer to engaging in addictive behavior because these thoughts represent a focus on action, rather than on mere contemplation of the desired effects of the addiction.

When automatic thoughts are activated, they are often accompanied by *urges and cravings*. Urges and cravings are experienced as strong physical sensations, similar to hunger or thirst. According to A. T. Beck et al. (1993), "Craving refers to a desire for the drug, whereas the term urge is applied to the internal pressure or mobilization to act on the craving.... In short, a craving is associated with wanting and an urge with doing" (p. 31). However, this distinction between urges and cravings is subtle, and the terms are used synonymously in CTAGs. People vary in the extent to which they experience urges and cravings. While freely engaging in addictive behavior, people rarely experience significant cravings. During withdrawal from many types of substances, the strength of urges and cravings escalates. Group members initially abstaining from substance use may experience severe cravings because they may continue to think about using drugs while resisting the desire to do so.

The likelihood that a person succumbs to urges and cravings and engages in addictive behavior depends, in part, on a third type of unhelpful cognition. *Facilitating thoughts* are cognitions that serve as permission to engage in addictive behavior. Examples of facilitating thoughts include "Liquor won't hurt me," "I'll stop after tonight," and "It's only one cigarette." At times, facilitating thoughts can be expressed as denial, minimization, or rationalization (Rotgers & Nguyen, 2006). Stronger facilitating thoughts lower the person's tolerance for urges and cravings and increase the likelihood that the person will engage in addictive behavior. After giving themselves permission to use, patients with addictions focus on *instrumental strategies* (i.e., action plans) in order to do what is necessary in order to engage in the addictive behavior. Instrumental strategies represent an important behavioral component of this cognitive model. Examples of instrumental strategies include keeping the refrigerator stocked with beer, driving to a convenience store, calling a dealer, or driving to a casino or strip club. *Continued use, lapse,* or *relapse* refers to the actual engagement

in the addictive behavior. Such behavior may range from a brief, spontaneous slip (e.g., one beer or cigarette) to lengthy binges. A lapse may become
a trigger in and of itself for future use and full relapse if it leads to the belief
that abstinence is unattainable.

Research designed to test aspects of this basic cognitive model of addiction has confirmed that patients with addictions indeed endorse anticipatory expectancies, relief-oriented expectancies, and facilitating thoughts to
a greater degree than people who do not struggle with addictions and that
these cognitions diminish with cognitive therapy (e.g., Hautekeete, Cousin,
& Graziani, 1999; Tison & Hautekeete, 1998). Furthermore, all of the
constructs in this model can be addressed directly using cognitive therapy.
Specifically, cognitive therapists can work with patients to reduce the likelihood that they will encounter a trigger that puts them at risk for engaging
in addictive behavior. In addition, they can help patients acquire strategies
for identifying, evaluating, and modifying outcome expectancies, automatic thoughts, and facilitating thoughts that arise in response to a trigger.
Cognitive therapy for addictions also allows patients to develop strategies
for coping with urges and cravings. Strategies to achieve these aims are
described at length in Part II.

Additional Cognitive Behavioral Constructs

Although anticipatory expectancies, relief-oriented expectancies, and
facilitating thoughts are the central cognitive constructs in the proximal
situational cognitive model of addiction, a few other relevant constructs
have received attention in the empirical literature and have relevance for
the understanding of the unfolding of addictive behavior in response to a
trigger. For example, many other cognitive behavioral models of addiction
emphasize the roles of coping and self-efficacy in affecting the likelihood
that a person will relapse (e.g., Marlatt & Witkiewitz, 2005; Monti et al.,
2002; Niaura et al., 1988). *Coping* is defined as "the thoughts and behaviors used to manage the internal and external demands of situations that
are appraised as stressful" (Folkman & Moskowitz, 2004, p. 745). *Self-
efficacy* is defined as a person's expectation that he or she can successfully
execute a desired behavior (Bandura, 1977).

Although self-efficacy can also be viewed as a distal background factor
that captures the degree to which people generally believe they can exert
desired effects on their environment, it is considered a proximal situational
variable in this model because it pertains to the degree to which people
believe they can exert desired behaviors in response to a specific cue or trigger. When a person encounters a trigger, he or she must implement a coping
response in order to avoid a lapse. If the coping response is successful, the
person's self-efficacy is increased, outcome expectancies about the positive

effects of the addiction are weakened, and the chances of a future lapse are lessened. However, if the coping response is unsuccessful, the person's self-efficacy decreases, outcome expectancies about the positive effects of the addiction are strengthened, and the chances of a future lapse are increased (cf. Brandon et al., 2004). In fact, empirical research has demonstrated that people who "feel like giving up" after a lapse in abstinence from smoking, an inclination that reflects low self-efficacy, are at an increased likelihood to move rapidly toward a second lapse (Shiffman, Hickcox, et al., 1996) and that self-efficacy predicts abstinence 3 months after the termination of treatment (Goldbeck, Myatt, & Aitchison, 1997).

Figure 2.3 displays the manner in which coping and self-efficacy apply to A. T. Beck et al.'s (1993) basic cognitive model of addiction. We view coping and self-efficacy as variables that have the potential to impact the entire cognitive behavioral sequence that leads to addictive behavior, and their impact is represented by the large downward arrow. In other words, effective coping and high self-efficacy can reduce the ease with which outcome expectancies, automatic thoughts, and facilitating thoughts are activated, as well as the strength of these cognitions and the urges and cravings experienced by the individual. Conversely, ineffective coping and low self-efficacy can increase the ease with which addiction-related cognitions are activated and the strength of these cognitions, urges, and cravings. It follows then, that intervening at the level of coping and self-efficacy could have a widespread ripple effect by influencing many of the cognitions and behaviors captured in the basic cognitive model.

Empirical research conducted over the past two decades has identified another important cognitive construct at work in addictions—an *attentional bias* toward addiction-related cues (see Bruce & Jones, 2006; Field & Cox, 2008; Field, Mogg, & Bradley, 2006, for reviews). An attentional bias occurs when patients with addictions detect cues that remind them of the addiction more quickly than they detect neutral, or unrelated stimuli. In many instances, the addicted individual fixates on or ruminates upon these cues, unable to direct his or her attention to a healthier focus and thereby increasing urges and cravings. Our group calls this phenomenon *attentional fixation*; others have referred to it as *cue fascination* (Sarnecki, Traynor, & Clune, 2008). Unlike the other cognitive constructs described in this chapter, attentional biases are not characterized by a specific content, but instead they depict a style of processing information. In other words, the expectancies, automatic thoughts, and facilitating thoughts capture *what* a person with an addiction is thinking, whereas an attentional bias characterizes *how* he or she is thinking.

According to Field and Cox (2008), attentional biases work through the activation of another expectancy—the expectation that the person has access to the object of one's addiction or can otherwise act on the

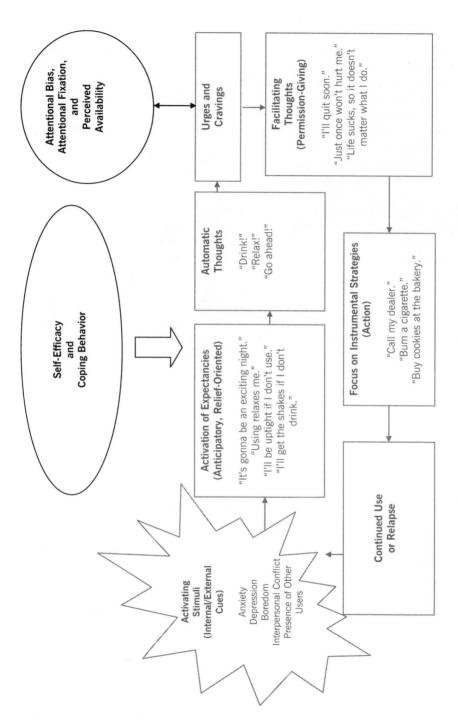

FIGURE 2.3. Proximal situational cognitive model of addiction.

addiction. For example, a person with an alcohol addiction experiences attentional biases toward alcohol-related cues when she believes that alcohol is readily available to her. A person with a gambling addiction experiences an attentional bias toward gambling-related cues when he believes he can easily travel to a casino. The link between addiction-related cues and the expectancy of availability initially develop through classical conditioning; that is, through repeated experiences, the person learns that the cue is associated with the availability of the addiction. Over time, the cue acquires strong motivational properties, and it becomes particularly salient when it is encountered because it is so "wanted" by the individual (Robinson & Berridge, 1993).

A key finding from research on addiction-related attentional biases is that there is a bidirectional relation between these biases and urges and cravings (e.g., Field & Eastwood, 2005). That is, when patients with an addiction detect an addiction-related cue, they experience a subsequent increase in urges and cravings. When they experience an increase in urges and cravings, they are more likely to detect and fixate on addiction-related cues. This bidirectional relation is captured in the right-most circle in Figure 2.3. According to this conceptualization of attentional biases, urges and cravings will be reduced when the individual can direct his or her attention away from addiction-related cues. CTAGs offer an array of strategies for doing just this, ranging from cognitive interventions to help patients evaluate the benefits and detriments of focusing on addiction-related cues (e.g., advantages–disadvantages analysis) to behavioral strategies that patients can use to distract themselves from addiction-related cues (see Chapter 8).

Distal Background Factors

To this point, we have proposed a cognitive model of addiction that accounts for the cognitive and behavioral processes at work when a person is faced with a trigger. Together, these processes increase or decrease the likelihood that the person will engage in addictive behavior in any one instance. However, these situational cognitive behavioral processes do not operate in isolation from an individual's personal history and unique constellation of vulnerability factors. For example, a person who struggles with addiction but who is free from other psychiatric problems may be able to deal more effectively with anticipatory expectancies, relief-oriented expectancies, and facilitating thoughts than a person who carries multiple psychiatric diagnoses. According to our model, the presence of one or more psychiatric disorders confers a nonspecific vulnerability for the activation of unhelpful addiction-related cognitions, which will in turn increase the likelihood of continued use, a lapse, or relapse. In the following section, we describe the cognitive–developmental model of addiction, first presented by Liese and

Franz (1996), which captures the formative experiences and fundamental beliefs that underlie addictive behavior. Subsequently, we identify other constructs that empirical research has identified as conferring additional vulnerability for engaging in addictive behaviors.

Cognitive–Developmental Model of Addiction

According to the cognitive–developmental model of addiction (Liese & Franz, 1996; see Figure 2.4), two main constructs set the stage for addictive behavior to occur: (1) environmental factors that provide an opportunity for learning, in the form of early experiences and exposure to addictive behavior; and (2) long-standing beliefs about the self, world, and the future, as well as beliefs about the addiction itself. *Early experiences* contribute to the development of basic beliefs about the self, world, and future. Significant or repetitive negative experiences put a person at risk for developing maladaptive or unhelpful beliefs, which in turn predispose him or her to develop mental health problems and addictive disorders. For example, a young girl who endures repeated sexual abuse may develop the belief that others cannot be trusted and later go on to develop significant problems with depression, anxiety, and interpersonal functioning. She might cope with these problems by drinking and using drugs. Although the identification of negative formative experiences that contribute to the development of maladaptive or unhelpful beliefs is a central activity in cognitive therapy, it is also important to recognize any positive formative experiences, as they could contribute to the development of beliefs that are associated with hope and resiliency.

Basic beliefs are beliefs about the self, world, and/or the future that can predispose a person to (or protect a person from) aversive emotional experiences, such as depression, guilt, anxiety, anger, loneliness, or boredom. According to Liese and Franz (1996), basic beliefs usually fall into one of two main domains. *Lovability* beliefs speak to a person's perception of connectedness, self-worth, and ability to maintain intimacy, whereas *adequacy* beliefs speak to a person's perception of competence, success, and autonomy. Maladaptive or unhelpful beliefs in both of these domains have been associated with clinical presentations such as depression, anxiety disorders, and personality disorders (A. T. Beck & Alford, 2009; Clark & Beck, 2010; A. T. Beck, Freeman, Davis, & Associates, 2004). However, basic beliefs can also affect the degree to which outcome expectancies and facilitating thoughts are activated, as well as the strength of a person's self-efficacy. It is not difficult to imagine that a person with a belief that she is unlovable would anticipate getting great relief from her emotional pain by engaging in addictive behavior, and that she would readily give herself permission to engage in addictive behavior because she does not believe

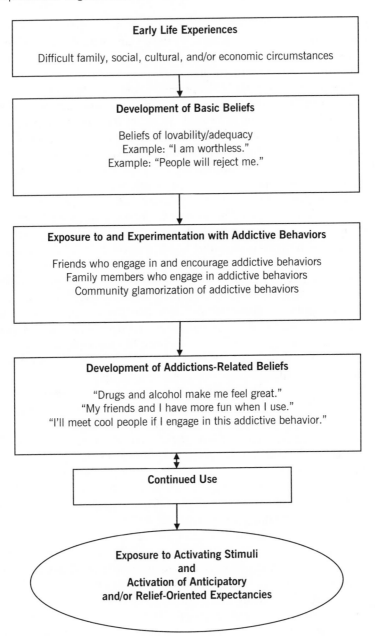

FIGURE 2.4. Cognitive–developmental model of addiction. Adapted from Liese and Franz (1996). Copyright 1996 by The Guilford Press. Adapted by permission.

anyone would care. Conversely, a person who holds the belief that he is incompetent might have very little self-efficacy and would readily give himself permission to engage in addictive behavior with the rationale that there is no point in trying to overcome it.

Although negative early life experiences and the presence of maladaptive or unhelpful basic beliefs increase the likelihood of addictive behavior in this model, they cannot fully explain addictions, as many people who have negative early life experiences and maladaptive basic beliefs do not have a problem with addictions. According to the cognitive–developmental model of addiction, two additional factors that have specific relevance to addictions must be in place. First, most people with addictions had *exposure to and experimentation with addictive behaviors* prior to having a full-fledged addictive disorder. Research shows that people who were exposed to addictive behavior in the home, such as when a parent drank or used drugs, are at an increased likelihood to develop an addictive disorder themselves (Anda et al., 2002; Merikangas, Dierker, & Szatmari, 1998). Other people with addictions were not exposed to addictive behavior in the home, but they began to experiment with addictive behaviors like drinking alcohol, smoking cigarettes, and/or using drugs during their adolescence and young adulthood. The frequency and degree of experimentation is often influenced by a person's basic beliefs. For example, youth who are formulating basic beliefs that they are unlovable or incompetent may be particularly susceptible to peer pressure to engage in addictive behavior.

Second, people with addictions usually develop strong *addiction-related beliefs* as a result of their exposure to and early experimentation with addictive behavior. According to Liese and Franz (1996), beliefs that facilitate anticipatory expectations often occur early in the history of a person's addictive behavior, whereas beliefs that facilitate relief-oriented expectancies often emerge later in the history of a person's addictive behavior. Moreover, certain types of basic beliefs may make people particularly vulnerable to develop unhealthy addiction-related beliefs. For example, a young adult who is forming an unlovability basic belief may be particularly likely to believe that engaging in addictive behavior makes her "cool" or "part of the in crowd." These addiction-related beliefs form a reciprocal relationship with *continued use*. They facilitate continued use because the person believes that they are associated with positive outcomes (cf. Rotgers & Nguyen, 2006). Continued use, in turn, enhances these beliefs and makes them more salient and accessible. As Liese and Franz (1996) noted, people become "trapped in vicious circles of drug use and belief reinforcement that escalate their addictions" (p. 484).

Many of the same cognitive therapy strategies that can be used to address proximal situational cognitions (e.g., outcome expectancies) can also be used to address constructs in the cognitive–developmental model of addiction. Although no type of psychotherapy can erase a person's early experiences and previous exposure to and experimentation with addictive behaviors, basic beliefs and addiction-related beliefs are modifiable with standard cognitive therapy strategies. Moreover, cognitive therapy can help people formulate adaptive meanings associated with unfortunate early experiences.

Other Relevant Distal Background Factors

Figure 2.5 displays the part of our comprehensive cognitive model that focuses on distal background factors, which incorporates constructs from Liese and Frantz's (1996) cognitive–developmental model of addiction and includes additional constructs that the empirical literature has determined puts people at risk for addictive disorders. We propose that a host of biopsychosocial factors contribute to the development of maladaptive or unhelpful basic beliefs and addiction-related beliefs. Some of these factors are the environmental, or social, ones included in the cognitive–developmental model of addiction, such as early life experiences and exposure to and experimentation with addictive behaviors. Other social factors that make people vulnerable to engage in addictive behavior (or protect people from engaging in addictive behavior) reflect their current circumstances, such as the degree to which they have family/social support and the degree to which they have access to meaningful activities in which they can participate on a regular basis (Hawkins, Catalano, & Miller, 1992; Monti et al., 2002). Specifically, we propose that a social support network that is (1) composed of people who do not engage in addictive behavior, and/or (2) viewed as helpful decreases the likelihood that a person will engage in addictive behavior, whereas a social support network that is (1) composed of people who indeed engage in addictive behavior, and/or (2) viewed as unhelpful or intrusive increases the likelihood that a person will engage in problematic addictive behavior. Similarly, we view the availability of meaningful, non-addiction-related activities as decreasing the likelihood of engaging in problematic addictive behavior and the absence of such activities as increasing the likelihood of engaging in problematic addictive behavior.

In addition, there is much empirical literature suggesting that some types of addictive behaviors, such as alcohol and drug use, have a genetic component (e.g., Kreek, Nielsen, Butelman, & LaForge, 2005). In some cases, the genetic predisposition is for personality characteristics like impulsivity, risk taking, or novelty seeking. In other cases, the genetic predisposition might affect the likelihood of the development, maintenance, and/or exacerbation of the addiction itself, such as increased sensitivity to a drug's rewarding properties (Forbes et al., 2009) or even abnormalities in a drug's effects at receptor sites or rate of metabolism (Kreek et al., 2005). Although a person's

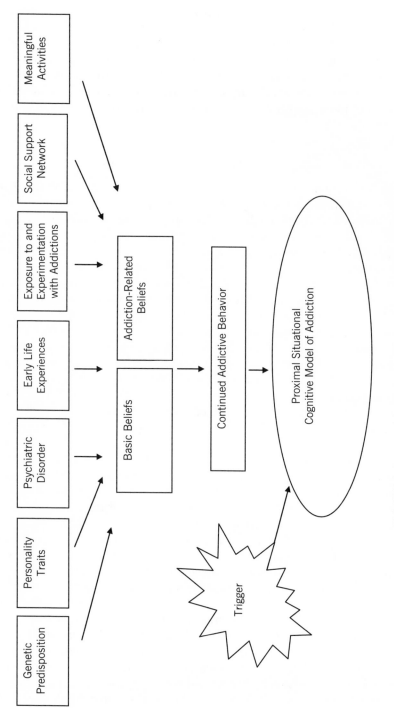

FIGURE 2.5. Distal background cognitive model of addiction.

genetic predisposition cannot be altered after the fact through any type of intervention, it can help the person understand his or her vulnerability to engage in addictive behavior and reduce the likelihood that a particular gene will be expressed. This knowledge allows him or her to be vigilant for instances in which this predisposition might manifest and to make healthy choices that minimize the expression of this genetic predisposition.

A potent biopsychosocial variable that can contribute to the likelihood of engaging in addictive behavior is a person's personality style. Personality characteristics have long been considered in cognitive models of addiction; in fact, A. T. Beck et al. (1993, p. 39) proposed several "predispositional characteristics" that make people vulnerable for addictions, including (1) sensitivity to unpleasant emotions; (2) inability to delay gratification; (3) poor techniques for controlling behavior; (4) automatic, nonreflective yielding to impulses; (5) excitement seeking and low tolerance for boredom; (6) low frustration tolerance; and (7) diminished future time perspective. In other words, people who have an acute sensitivity for reward and who consistently demonstrate behavioral undercontrol are, potentially, at risk for the development of an addictive disorder.

The personality trait that has perhaps received the most attention in the empirical literature is impulsivity. The collective body of research clearly demonstrates that, as a group, people with addictive disorders are more impulsive than people without addictive disorders (Moeller & Dougherty, 2002). Although most of us would easily be able to provide a definition of impulsivity when called upon to do so, the construct has been surprisingly difficult to operationalize in the scholarly literature (Enticott & Ogloff, 2006). Some scholars view impulsivity as a global personality trait (e.g., Dom, D'haene, Hulstijn, & Sabbe, 2006); others view it as a cognitive deficit (e.g., an inability to plan ahead; Whiteside & Lynam, 2001); and still others view it as a behavioral deficit (e.g., Perry & Carroll, 2008). In fact, there are *many* behavioral deficits that fall under the umbrella of impulsivity, including deficits in *response initiation* (i.e., responding before a stimulus is fully processed and evaluated), *response inhibition* (i.e., an inability to inhibit a response that has already been initiated), and *consequence sensitivity* (i.e., persistent responding despite negative consequences; Dougherty et al., 2009). One definition that sums up many of these features is "a predisposition to rapid, unplanned reactions to internal or external stimuli with diminished regard to the negative consequences of these reactions to the ... individual or others" (Potenza & Taylor, 2009, p. 714).

Not only do personality traits make people vulnerable to engage in addictive behavior and ultimately develop an addictive disorder, it is also likely that they influence the course of addictive disorders. Continuing with the example of impulsivity, it is logical to hypothesize that an impulsive person would quickly succumb to anticipatory and relief-oriented expectancies, as well as cling to facilitating thoughts at the expense of cognition that would deter him or her from engaging in addictive behavior (e.g., considering the long-term consequences of relapse). In addition, empirical research suggests that impulsivity increases the likelihood of relapse and decreases the likelihood that a person will stay in treatment (Moeller, Dougherty, et al., 2001). Thus, it is important to realize that personality traits like impulsivity cannot be viewed separately from the addictive behavior, as there is dynamic interplay between the two. There is even evidence for a bidirectional relation between personality factors and addictive behaviors; for example, it is likely that impulsivity becomes even more pronounced in people with alcohol dependence after chronic alcohol use (Lawrence, Luty, Bogdan, Sahakian, & Clark, 2009).

As referenced earlier in this chapter, another biopsychosocial factor that can increase the likelihood that a person will engage in addictive behavior and develop an addictive disorder is the presence of one or more psychiatric disorders. Specific types of psychiatric disorders that have the potential to increase the likelihood of addictive behavior include but are not limited to mood disorders (e.g., depression, bipolar disorder), anxiety disorders (e.g., panic disorder, social anxiety disorder), attention-deficit/ hyperactivity disorder, and Axis II disorders (e.g., borderline personality disorder, antisocial personality disorder). Research confirms that there are much higher rates of addictive behavior and addictive disorders in people with psychiatric disorders than in people without psychiatric disorders (cf. B. F. Grant et al., 2004; Swendsen et al., 2010). It is likely that psychiatric disorders confer vulnerability in many ways, such as by influencing the development of unhelpful basic beliefs and addiction-related beliefs, by increasing the likelihood that a person will experience stress or negative life events that could serve as triggers, and by decreasing self-efficacy and the execution of adaptive coping behavior when a person is faced with a decision of whether to engage in addictive behavior. Conversely, it is also likely that addictions, in turn, exacerbate the expression of psychiatric symptoms (cf. Flores, 2007).

It is important to keep in mind that the distal background factors described in this section, as well as other potential distal background factors, are not entirely independent. For example, certain personality traits, like impulsivity, increase the likelihood of a range of psychiatric disorders, not only addictive disorders (Moeller, Barratt, Dougherty, Schmitz, & Swann, 2001). The strength and composition of a person's social support network can influence the degree to which a person is exposed to and experiments with addictive behaviors, and conversely, exposure to and experimentation with addictive behaviors might begin to affect a person's social support network (Hawkins et al., 1992; Kobus & Henry, 2010). Thus, it is important to keep in mind that the distal background factors are interrelated and, in many cases, likely exert bidirectional effects on one another.

Together, these distal background factors affect the development of basic beliefs about the self, world, and future, as well as addiction-related beliefs that set the stage for anticipatory and relief-oriented expectancies. Because basic beliefs can also affect the development of addiction-related beliefs, and addiction-related beliefs have the potential to entrench unhelpful basic beliefs, we also view these two constructs as interrelated. According to our theory, the activation of unhelpful basic beliefs and addiction-related beliefs facilitate continued addictive behavior. This entire model—the distal background factors, the basic and addiction-related beliefs, and continued use—create the context for the proximal situational factors to be put in motion when a person encounters a trigger and is faced with the decision of whether to engage in addictive behavior.

Although much of the CTAG is devoted to developing strategies to manage cognitions and behaviors that are specifically related to addictive behaviors, undoubtedly, group members will resonate with many of the other distal background factors, such as the presence of a psychiatric disorder or an unsatisfactory social support network. When group facilitators determine that such factors are relevant to the majority of group members and are contributing to their struggles in meeting their goals, they can use cognitive therapy strategies to address them and demonstrate to members the manner in which attention given to these areas will contribute to recovery. Examples of ways to integrate focus on such distal background factors are described in Part II.

SUMMARY

Our comprehensive cognitive model of addiction has integrated A. T. Beck et al.'s (1993) basic cognitive model of addiction, Liese and Franz's (1996) cognitive–developmental model of addiction, and additional constructs that research has shown to affect cognitive behavioral processes associated with addictive behaviors. In short, we propose that the variables included in the distal background model of addiction (i.e., distal background factors, basic beliefs, addiction-related beliefs) increase the likelihood that the proximal situational cognitive model of addiction (i.e., outcome expectancies, automatic thoughts, urges and cravings, facilitating thoughts, coping, self-efficacy, attentional biases; cf. Moos, 2007) will be activated when a person encounters a trigger (illustrated in the simplified Figure 2.1). Successful treatment of the person with an addictive disorder will address both the (1) cognitive, emotional, behavioral, and physiological events that occur in the time that he or she makes a decision to engage in addictive behavior; and (2) modifiable distal background factors and long-standing beliefs.

Although this model is comprehensive, it is also general in that it pertains to people with addictive disorders, as a group, rather than to any one individual. Each person will be uniquely characterized by his or her own profile of proximal and distal factors that contribute to his or her addictive behavior. As such, a critical component of the CTAG, as in any cognitive therapy protocol, is to complete a cognitive case conceptualization for each group member. The cognitive case conceptualization brings the comprehensive cognitive model of addiction to life for each individual group member and points to the most logical points of intervention that will ultimately help to reduce the likelihood of continued addictive behavior. We explain more about the process of cognitive case conceptualization in Chapter 5, and in Chapters 7 and 8, we illustrate the manner in which constructs from this model can be targeted in treatment. Throughout the volume, we use the terms *cognitive model* and *comprehensive cognitive model of addiction* interchangeably.

We believe that a sound understanding of this comprehensive cognitive model of addiction is crucial for clinicians who run CTAGs. It provides a context for both facilitators and group members to understand the factors that can account for the unfolding of an addictive disorder. The model provides a straightforward framework for the facilitators to describe the cognitive approach to addictions to group members. Group members, then, can use this knowledge to build an awareness of the processes at work when they are at risk for a lapse. The cliché, "knowledge is power," is relevant here—the more group members can put words to the cognitive and behavioral events that might facilitate addictive behavior, the more they can begin to recognize when they are falling into traps that can lead to a slip or a lapse. Although we view the comprehensive cognitive model of addiction as the cornerstone of the CTAG, it is also important for facilitators to be aware of other relevant theory that does not necessarily have its origins in the cognitive behavioral approach but that is significant in capturing the processes at work in group treatment for addictions. In the next chapter, we provide an overview of two additional theoretical perspectives—theory that is relevant to group process, and theory that is relevant to group members' readiness for change.

CHAPTER 3 | Theoretical Framework

Group Theory and the Stages-of-Change Model

An understanding of the comprehensive cognitive model of addiction, described in Chapter 2, is crucial for identifying the cognitive and behavioral factors that maintain each group member's addiction, as well as for deciding upon specific intervention strategies. However, it is only one part of the theoretical background necessary to run successful CTAGs. Facilitators must also be familiar with two other theoretical traditions: (1) theory associated with the implementation of group psychotherapy and group process (e.g., Yalom & Leszcz, 2005), and (2) theory associated with patients' readiness for change (e.g., Prochaska & DiClemente, 2005).

A strong grasp of the theoretical framework that underlies the successful implementation of group psychotherapy will allow facilitators to harness the power of group support and interaction. Failure to recognize this dynamic puts facilitators at risk of conducting a group that feels like a classroom, with little opportunity for interaction among group members. Groups conducted in this manner do not capitalize, then, on an important mechanism of change. A strong grasp of the theoretical framework that underlies patients' readiness for change will allow facilitators to tailor intervention strategies to meet the needs of group members. Patients with addictive disorders are often ambivalent about change, as, at times, they are reluctant to give up the perceived rewards associated with addictive behavior, and they view the road to recovery as one that is too difficult for them to tackle. Application of theory associated with group members' readiness for change will guide facilitators in selecting strategies to motivate group members who are ambivalent and to maximize the commitment of group members who are ready to take action. In this chapter, we describe both theoretical approaches.

GROUP PSYCHOTHERAPY

There is no question that facilitators of successful psychotherapy groups devote much attention to group process and identify ways to use group process as a vehicle of change for group members. According to the Clinical Practice Guidelines for Group Psychotherapy (Bernard et al., 2008), *group process* is defined as "what happens in the group, especially in terms of the development and evolution of patterns of relationships between and among group members" (p. 496). In this section, we consider the therapeutic principles that underlie effective group psychotherapy that have been identified and developed by a pioneer group therapist, Irvin Yalom. During this discussion, we draw on the work of Bieling et al. (2006), who have thoughtfully considered the manner in which Yalom's principles apply specifically to cognitive behavioral group psychotherapy.

Figure 3.1 displays the 11 primary factors that account for the effectiveness of group therapy, as described by Yalom and Leszcz (2005). For example, in every group session, there is an opportunity for the *instillation of hope* and the *imparting of information*. At times, these processes are realized when facilitators present group members with information, called *psychoeducation*, about addictions in general, the efficacy of cognitive therapy for addictions, and/or the cognitive model that underlies their problems (Bieling et al., 2006). This information allows group members to realize that many others have been treated successfully with cognitive therapy in the past and that there is a logical framework to understand their life problems. The installation of hope and the imparting of information also occur when group members give advice, suggestions, and guidance to one another. In many instances, new group members develop a sense of optimism that they can change when the gains made by seasoned group members are showcased.

A sense of *universality* is reinforced when people with a similar problem come together, share their stories, and recognize the similarities they have with one another. According to Yalom and Leszcz (2005), group members often experience a pronounced sense of relief when they realize they are not alone or unique in their struggles. Many patients with addictions develop basic beliefs about themselves when they are faced with the consequences of their addictive behavior, such as "I'm a failure," "I'm a burden," and/or "I'm broken." Realizing that others have endured similar struggles and seeing examples of others who have successfully overcome their addiction provide important pieces of evidence that are contrary to these beliefs, allowing group members to consider entertaining a different set of beliefs that is more likely to promote sobriety and good mental health.

Group members have many opportunities for *altruism* when they assist other group members in the application of cognitive and behavioral

- **Instillation of hope:** Group members develop optimism that treatment will be helpful for them by learning about the effectiveness of the group and by hearing about other group members' positive outcomes.

- **Imparting information:** Group members learn new information through didactic instruction by the facilitators and through advice given by fellow group members.

- **Universality:** Group members realize that others are struggling with similar difficulties, in contrast to their initial view that their problems are unique.

- **Altruism:** Group members take opportunities to help one another and benefit from this process by deriving a sense of value for their contributions.

- **Imitative behavior:** Group members learn by observing the behaviors of other group members and of the facilitator(s).

- **Development of socializing techniques:** Group members acquire and practice social skills.

- **Interpersonal learning:** Group members learn, through their interactions in the group, about their own interpersonal styles and the impact they have on others and use these insights to change their own interpersonal patterns.

- **Group cohesiveness:** Group members experience acceptance, trust, belongingness, and support from one another.

- **Existential factors:** Group members deal with issues related to the human condition, including isolation, mortality, freedom, responsibility, and the search for meaning.

- **Catharsis:** Group members share painful experiences and emotional reactions in the group setting.

- **The corrective recapitulation of the primary family group:** Group members engage in the same interpersonal behaviors in which they engaged with primary family members, and they have the opportunity to have corrective experiences that resolve long-standing issues related to the family.

FIGURE 3.1. Yalom and Leszcz's (2005) therapeutic factors. At times, group psychotherapy experts refer to 12 or 13, rather than 11, therapeutic factors relevant to the implementation of group psychotherapy (e.g., Bernard et al., 2008). Research into these therapeutic factors is ongoing and evolving, becoming more nuanced over time. However, these 11 factors are considered to be the consistent core characteristics (Molyn Leszcz, personal communication, June 27, 2011). Sources for this figure include Yalom and Leszcz (2005); Bernard et al. (2008); and Bieling, McCabe, and Antony (2006).

strategies to managing their life problems. Of course, the group member who receives this assistance benefits greatly, in that he or she will gain a unique perspective on his or her problems and the implementation of cognitive and behavioral strategies. However, Yalom and Leszcz (2005) also acknowledged the powerful effects that altruism can have on the person who provides the assistance. Many group members carry the belief that they do not have anything valuable to offer others. Thus, the opportunity to provide assistance to others provides evidence contrary to this belief and contributes to the development of a belief of self-worth and value.

Imitative behavior occurs when group members model their behavior on the behavior of others, which is a principle that Yalom and Leszcz (2005) believe is a particularly potent factor in groups, like the CTAG, that have a single focus. Thus, facilitators seize the opportunity for imitative behavior by encouraging group members to practice using the cognitive and behavioral strategies with one another, which allows them to learn vicariously to apply these strategies (Bieling et al., 2006). It is also important for facilitators to keep this principle in mind regarding their own behavior as they conduct sessions. Facilitators often encounter challenging moments as they conduct sessions, such as instances in which one group member's behavior has the potential to be disruptive to others, or when it is clear that most group members are not responding to the particular intervention that they are attempting to implement. In these instances, facilitators address these challenges using the same cognitive and behavioral strategies that they are imparting to the group. For example, they check out the accuracy of assumptions they are making regarding the group process that they are observing, taking care not to act on the assumptions until they are verified. They might also use the social skills they are coaching group members to acquire. When facilitators model the cognitive and behavioral strategies to address an issue that arises in session, they take care to ensure that group members recognize that they are using these strategies and to consider the manner in which these strategies generalize to their own lives.

Socializing techniques are developed in each group session through active interaction with one another, and they provide the opportunity for group members to acquire basic social skills that are expected to enhance their relationships outside of session (Bieling et al., 2006). The more a person has participated in a psychotherapy group, the more he or she is likely to develop the abilities to be responsive, empathetic, and nonjudgmental toward others (Yalom & Leszcz, 2005). Moreover, the presence of tension between group members allows a rare opportunity for group members to develop effective conflict resolution skills that can be applied to manage tension in their relationships outside of the group setting. As is discussed in greater length in Chapter 8, many patients with addictions have significant disturbances in their close relationships, and the development of social skills can serve as an important vehicle in repairing these relationships. As a result of the practice of these social skills, group members also achieve *interpersonal learning*, which occurs when they begin to recognize the impact of their own interpersonal style on others. This information can help group members develop healthier and more accurate beliefs about themselves and others, and it also allows them to hone their practice of social skills as they become more interpersonally effective.

Group cohesiveness, also called *cohesion* in the empirical literature, refers to "the emotional bonds among group members for each other and a shared commitment to the group and its primary task" (Bernard et al., 2008, p. 497) and is often regarded as synonymous with the therapeutic relationship in a group setting (Burlingame, Fuhriman, & Johnson, 2002). According to Yalom and Leszcz (2005), there are many components of group cohesiveness, including the relationships between the facilitators and the group members, the relationships among the various group members, and the relationships between each group member and the group as a whole. A high level of group cohesiveness is associated with a sense of warmth, comfort, belongingness, acceptance, commitment, and value. Research shows that group cohesiveness has a moderate association with patient outcome ($r = .25$) and that this association becomes even stronger when facilitators specifically attend to group cohesion during sessions (Burlingame, McClendon, & Alonso, 2011). Although Yalom and Leszcz regarded group cohesiveness as a therapeutic mechanism in its own right, they also viewed it as the basis from which the other therapeutic principles emerge (cf. Bernard et al., 2008). CTAG facilitators monitor cohesiveness throughout the life of the group, and they encourage group members to make overt expressions of encouragement, support, and trust in order to build cohesion among group members. Strategic decisions made in session in order to foster group cohesiveness include providing a safe environment for self-disclosure, promoting interaction and support among the group members, highlighting specific similarities among group members, encouraging the sharing of information, and attending to group process in the present (Bieling et al., 2006).

Throughout their participation in group, group members address *existential factors* when they deal with issues related to the human condition, including isolation, mortality, freedom, responsibility, and the search for meaning. All of these existential factors are relevant to understanding, modifying, and taking responsibility for the effects of each group member's basic and addiction-related beliefs and self-defeating addictive behavior.

Bieling et al. (2006) regarded two of Yalom's factors as being less relevant than the others to cognitive behavioral groups, in part because aspects of these tenets are not central to cognitive behavioral theory. First, *catharsis* is not always emphasized in cognitive behavioral therapies as a strategic process in and of itself. Of course, most, if not all, clinicians would argue that group members need to share information about themselves, especially information that has the potential to be embarrassing, painful, or distressing, in order to maximize the use of group support. We agree that, in the successful CTAG, most group members will speak candidly about their life problems. They may even feel a sense of catharsis after doing so. However, in cognitive therapy, disclosure of painful or distressing information is seen as only the first of many steps. In addition to giving patients space to provide such disclosure in a warm, inviting environment, cognitive therapists work with their patients to (1) conceptualize their problems from a cognitive and behavioral framework, and (2) apply one or more cognitive or behavioral strategies in order to promote active coping, problem solving, and/or acceptance. Thus, a balance that must be achieved by any cognitive therapist, including CTAG facilitators, is to allow for adequate disclosure of life problems and emotional distress while providing a framework for the patient to recognize an unhelpful style of coping and develop a more helpful style of coping.

A second factor that Bieling et al. (2006) regard as less relevant to cognitive behavioral groups is the *corrective recapitulation of the primary family group*, largely because cognitive therapy is focused on current life problems rather than the "working through" of early developmental experiences. Although early developmental experiences might be recognized and discussed in order for group members to recognize the role these formative experiences played in the development of their addictive behavior, we agree that the main purpose of the CTAG is generally not to "work through" these issues. Rather, group members recognize triggers for current urges, cravings, and unpleasant emotional experiences in light of these formative experiences and develop strategies for coping. However, we recognize that problematic styles of interacting with others and managing relationships, which in many cases reflect patterns enacted in early familial relationships, eventually become evident during the course of participation in any group. The CTAG offers many strategies for addressing these interpersonal styles, such as the opportunity for group members to provide feedback on these interpersonal styles, learn information about basic social skills, identify and modify cognitions that have the potential to interfere with the successful application of social skills, and practice the social skills (see Chapters 7 and 8). These strategies harness many of Yalom and Leszcz's (2005) therapeutic factors already discussed in this chapter, including the imparting of information, altruism, the development of socializing techniques, interpersonal learning, and imitative behavior. The support and feedback shared among group members during a discussion on this topic could, in turn, enhance group cohesiveness.

The most important point to keep in mind is that cognitive therapy is a treatment that balances a focus on the *process* of therapy (e.g., development of the therapeutic relationship; see Gilbert & Leahy, 2007; Wenzel, Brown, & Karlin, 2011) with the application of specific *techniques*, defined as "the commonly understood learning tools and strategies by which patients are educated about their disorder, or are taught to examine their behaviors, thoughts, and feelings, and any strategy designed to change this cognitive-behavioral system" (Bieling at al., 2006, p. 19). In the CTAG, specifically, facilitators are mindful of Yalom and Leszcz's (2005) therapeutic factors as they conduct the group, taking care to balance interventions that promote group cohesiveness with interventions that promote cognitive and behavioral change in group members. Because cognitive therapists aim to teach their patients the underlying principles of and rationale for cognitive therapy, there are several instances in any one CTAG in which facilitators will provide psychoeducation, or focus on one particular group member in order to illustrate an important principle that will be relevant to all group members. However, CTAG facilitators recognize that there is much more to group cognitive therapy than teaching, and they provide a safe environment in order for interactions between group members to provide, perhaps, the most powerful demonstration of these principles in action. We encourage interested readers to consult the works of Bernard et al. (2008), Flores (2007), and Yalom and Leszcz (2005) for additional consideration of group process and strategies for facilitating it.

READINESS FOR CHANGE

The transtheoretical model of behavior change (TTM) was developed to capture the dynamic course of an individual's process of change in treatment. Two main components of the TTM that are relevant to the conduct of CTAGs are (1) *stages of change*, which reflect the degree to which a person is ready to make positive behavioral changes in his or her life, and (2) *processes of change*, which are the strategies by which the person achieves lasting behavioral change (Prochaska & DiClemente, 2005). It has been proposed that treatment is most effective when the strategies selected by a therapist match with a patient's stage of change (e.g., Norcross et al., 2011).

Figure 3.2 summarizes the stages of change, as specified in the TTM: (1) precontemplation, (2) contemplation, (3) preparation, (4) action, and (5) maintenance. Our experience in conducting CTAGs is that consideration of each group member's stage of change is imperative. According to Norcross et al. (2011), many clinicians mistakenly assume that their patients are in the action stage, and they apply intervention strategies that are not appropriate. In fact, they estimated that about 40% of new patients are in the precontemplation stage, 40% are in the contemplation stage, and only 20% are prepared to take action. In many cases, the patients who are not prepared for action drop out of treatment because the clinician does not actively engage them in the decision-making process, or in weighing the advantages and disadvantages of giving up their addiction. Thus, recognizing a patient's stage of change and engaging him or her in light of that stage of change is crucial.

- **Precontemplation:** The person is either unaware of the nature and extent of his or her problematic behavior or is unwilling to make a change.
- **Contemplation:** The person recognizes that his or her behavior is problematic and is weighing the advantages and disadvantages of changing the problematic behavior. However, he or she continues to be swayed by perceived positive consequences of the problematic behavior and/or perceived enormity of the time, energy, cost, and loss associated with changing.
- **Preparation:** The person has resolved the decision-making process from the contemplation stage and has expressed a readiness to change in the near future (e.g., within the next month). The person may have made small behavioral changes in order to begin addressing the problematic behavior.
- **Action:** The person has implemented a change plan, is engaged in active coping, and is making more overt behavioral changes.
- **Maintenance:** The person has sustained meaningful behavioral change for at least 6 months and is focused on relapse prevention and on consolidating the gains made in treatment.

FIGURE 3.2. The TTM's stages of change. Sources: DiClemente and Prochaska (1998); Norcross, Krebs, and Prochaska (2011); Prochaska and DiClemente (2005).

Research shows that there is a moderate effect size (i.e., $d = 0.46$) for the association between stages of change and psychotherapy outcome, such that patients who are in the preparation and action stages of change tend to make more gains in treatment than patients in the precontemplation and the contemplation stages of change (Norcross et al., 2011). For example, one study that examined smokers with coronary artery disease found verified cessation rates after 12 months in 43% patients who presented for treatment in the action stage, 24% of patients who presented for treatment in the contemplation stage, and 14% of the patients who presented for treatment in the precontemplation stage (Ockene et al., 1992). The collective body of research suggests that patients will have the most success in treatment if they are in the preparation or action stages of change, which suggests that it would behoove clinicians to identify patients who are in the precontemplation and contemplation stages of change and implement strategies to address their ambivalence and help them move through the stages. Principles of motivational interviewing (Miller & Rollnick, 2002), which are incorporated into many other cognitive behavioral treatments for addiction (e.g., L. C. Sobell & Sobell, 2011), would be logical to implement as facilitators work with group members who are in the early stages of change.

The notion of stages of change can be applied to the understanding of the clinical presentations of each of the cases presented in Chapter 1. Dave presented for treatment in the precontemplation stage of change. He clearly stated that he is attending the group because his probation officer required it, and on most occasions, he indicates that he does not see his substance use as a problem, other than the fact that he lost his license. Michael, in contrast, is moving from the action stage of change to the maintenance stage of change. He has actively participated in the CTAG for the past 8 months, and, for the past 6 months, he has remained abstinent from extra-marital sexual activity, otherwise inappropriate relationships with other women, and pornography. Ellen is in the contemplation stage of change. Although she verbally expresses a commitment to modify her unhealthy eating habits, her verbal commitment has not translated to action, and she repeatedly engages in self-defeating behavior that distances her from her goals. Allison is moving from the preparation stage of change to the action stage of change. She has already significantly decreased the number of cigarettes she smokes, and she exhibits a strong motivation to achieve abstinence, both verbally and behaviorally. Finally, Brian represents the type of patient who "recycles" through various stages of change (cf. Norcross et al., 2011). Although, at times, he has demonstrated motivation for change and exhibited corresponding reductions in his gambling, he has relapsed on many occasions, including recently, bringing him back to the group. At present, he is dejected, unable to see how he can achieve his financial goals without gambling, and, therefore, unable to identify a specific change plan. Currently, Brian is best characterized as being in the contemplation stage of change.

The stages of change represent *when* people change, but it is the processes of change that represent *how* people change (Norcross et al., 2011). Figure 3.3 summarizes the 10 processes of change that are included in the TTM. Although cognitive therapists might use different language to describe the specific strategies implemented in any one session, the underlying principles are the same. For example, consciousness is raised in every single CTAG session because psychoeducation is provided about the cognitive model of addiction. Counterconditioning is achieved through almost all of the strategic interventions described in this volume, as group members learn the process of cognitive restructuring to replace unhelpful cognitions with more helpful, or balanced cognitions, and they also develop coping skills to replace problematic behaviors with more adaptive behaviors. Stimulus control often assumes a great deal of attention in CTAGs, as group members actively work to identify triggers and develop strategies for staying away from triggers and managing urges, cravings, and distress when an encounter with a trigger is unavoidable. Throughout the volume, we describe the manner in which the CTAG strategies are associated with these processes of change.

As stated previously, it has been suggested that the specific process of change selected depends on the individual patient's stage of change (e.g., Prochaska & DiClemente, 2005). For example, some research has found

- **Consciousness raising:** The process by which the person learns more about himself or herself and the causes, consequences, and cures for a problem behavior. This can often be achieved through psychoeducation and/or bibliotherapy.
- **Self liberation:** The process by which the person becomes aware of alternatives and makes more active choices in his or her life.
- **Social liberation:** The process by which the environment allows the person more choice.
- **Counterconditioning:** The process by which the person changes his or her responses to stimuli, substituting healthier behaviors for problem behaviors.
- **Stimulus control:** The process by which the person manages the triggers that prompt problem behavior.
- **Self-reevaluation:** The process by which the person assesses feelings and thoughts about him- or herself with and without the problem behavior.
- **Environmental reevaluation:** The process by which the person considers the social and physical impact of his or her problem behavior.
- **Contingency management:** The process by which the person makes changes by changing the contingencies in the environment (rewards/punishers).
- **Helping relationships:** The process by which the person uses relationships in his or her life to garner support for behavior change. Helping relationships include those with others in the person's social support system, with the therapist, and with others in a self-help group or group therapy.
- **Dramatic relief:** The process by which the person experiences and expresses affect about his or her problems and proposed solutions.

FIGURE 3.3. The TTM's processes of change. Sources: Norcross, Krebs, and Prochaska (2011); Prochaska and DiClemente (1982); Prochaska and Velicer (1997).

that cognitive and affective strategies (e.g., consciousness raising, self-reevaluation) are particularly helpful in moving patients from the precontemplation to the contemplation stage so that these patients can identify benefits of participating in treatment and envision how they would feel about themselves if they were to change, whereas behavioral change strategies (e.g., counterconditioning, stimulus control) are most appropriate during the action and maintenance stages (e.g., Rosen, 2000). Of course, it is difficult to select the "perfect" strategic intervention during any one group session, as group members who participate in the CTAG will be in different stages of change, and in many cases, disparate strategies cannot be implemented simultaneously. Nevertheless, facilitators can keep these guiding principles in mind as they develop conceptualizations of each group member's individual clinical presentation as well as the conceptualization of the group as a whole and select strategic therapeutic interventions (see Chapter 5 for more information).

SUMMARY

The CTAG is a group psychotherapy approach to treat addictive behavior that has firm roots in three theoretical traditions: (1) cognitive theory (described in Chapter 2), (2) theory related to group process, and (c) aspects of the TTM. CTAG facilitators keep guiding principles in mind from all three theoretical frameworks in order to balance attention to group cohesiveness with the application of change-based therapeutic strategies, to conceptualize the clinical presentations of individual group members and the group as a whole, and to tailor process- and change-based interventions so that they are relevant to group members in different stages of change.

Although this might seem like a tall order, there are many aspects of the CTAG that facilitate the successful translation of these theories to clinical practice. As is described in Chapter 4, any one CTAG is typically run by two co-facilitators, which increases the likelihood that, between the two of them, important manifestations of these theories are recognized in interactions with each group member. In addition, a key tenet of cognitive therapy is collaboration, which means that the decision to pursue any one therapeutic intervention is made by the facilitators and group members, together. Thus, if facilitators are moving toward selecting a therapeutic intervention that fails to recognize when an important aspect of one of these theories is at work, they will receive feedback from group members that will help them to make adjustments.

In the next chapter, we provide an overview of the CTAG, illustrating the main participants in and components of the CTAG. The subsequent chapters describe the clinical implementation of the specific CTAG components. Throughout the volume, we link the theoretical tenets described in Chapter 2 and this chapter with the implementation of specific therapeutic strategies, which will allow readers to understand the manner in which theory translates to clinical application in the group treatment of patients with addictive disorders.

CHAPTER 4 | Overview of the Cognitive Therapy Addictions Group (CTAG)

CTAGs are active, directive, semistructured psychotherapy groups designed to help individuals overcome addictive behavior. Figure 4.1 displays the main characteristics of this treatment approach. Groups are facilitated by mental health professionals who apply, model, and teach the concepts and strategies of cognitive therapy while simultaneously facilitating group cohesiveness and support. CTAGs are compatible with most existing addiction treatment modalities (e.g., 12-step programs). They usually meet for 90-minute sessions once per week, although sessions can be as long as 2 hours (Bieling et al., 2006). Groups can either be small (e.g., 5 to 6 members) or large (e.g., 10 to 12 members) and can include people with various addictions at various stages in the change process. Facilitators use this diversity to illustrate commonalities among an array of addictive behaviors, highlight successful application of cognitive and behavioral strategies in seasoned group members, and provide a context of support and encouragement for new group members or group members who continue to engage in addictive behavior.

A key feature of cognitive therapy, including the CTAG, is that it is *collaborative*, which means that group members and facilitators work together actively and as equal partners to create a stimulating learning environment and to solve problems. Although all group members are encouraged to participate in sessions, it is understood that some people are not comfortable talking in a group, and these members' wishes regarding participation are respected. Some group members even report that their most important learning experiences in CTAGs are vicarious, as they quietly listen to others deal with their addictions and observe the manner in which they apply cognitive and behavioral strategies to their lives. Thus, group members

- Sessions are active, directed, and structured.
- The group is usually facilitated by two mental health professionals (e.g., psychologists, psychiatrists, social workers, certified drug and alcohol counselors, psychiatric nurses, certified counselors).
- The group is compatible with other addiction treatment modalities (e.g., 12-step programs).
- Sessions last 90 minutes to 2 hours.
- The group can be small (e.g., 5 to 6 members) or large (e.g., 10 to 12 members).
- The group includes members with a variety of different addictions at various stages in the change process.
- The group is collaborative, educational, and supportive.
- The group is open and accepts new members on a rolling basis.
- Facilitators use a combination of Socratic questioning and didactic presentation of information.
- Goals of the group include (1) modification of addictive behavior, (2) development of cognitive and behavioral coping strategies, and (3) fostering of group support and cohesiveness.
- Facilitators meet with potential group members prior to their first group session.
- Patients are appropriate for the CTAG if they have the capability to understand the content that is discussed and interact appropriately with the facilitators and other group members, and they are addressing problems that have the potential to limit their participation in group in other treatment settings.
- The group follows a standard but flexible session structure.

FIGURE 4.1. Basic characteristics of CTAGs.

are encouraged to participate actively, with active participation defined as attention to, tracking of, and consideration of group discussion in addition to verbal contributions. Collaboration is also demonstrated when facilitators work together with group members to make decisions about how to spend their time (e.g., the topic to be covered in a particular session) and the kind of work to do in between sessions. This sort of collaboration not only encourages active participation, but it also shows that group members' opinions are valuable and important.

Most of the time, CTAG facilitators engage group members in the process of *Socratic questioning*. Socratic questioning involves the use of focused questioning and reflective responses to help group members to critically evaluate their cognitions and behaviors and discover their own answers to important questions and problems. This approach to treatment allows group members to actively apply cognitive strategies and problem-solving skills, which increases the likelihood that they will be able to apply such skills to problems that arise in their daily lives. However, at other times the facilitator may act as a teacher, educating group members about addictions, cognitive therapy, and coping strategies. In some instances, group members who have attended several sessions model the application of cognitive and behavioral strategies for new members. Although the "teaching" approach is very effective for presenting new material to group members, facilitators take care to limit the amount of didactic presentation of material in any one group session, as it is important for group members to view the treatment as psychotherapy and not simply as a "class."

It is most common for structured psychotherapy groups, particularly psychotherapy groups that use the cognitive behavioral approach, to start with a set number of members and to be closed to new members after they have begun (Bieling et al., 2006). In contrast, CTAGs are open-ended and ongoing; therefore, group members can seek help (i.e., come and go) when they need it, rather than waiting for the start of a new group. This open-ended nature enables CTAGs to be offered in a variety of treatment settings on an inpatient or outpatient basis, many of which serve patients who receive services for a short period of time or only on an occasional basis. Moreover, it allows patients to get as much treatment as they need, as some experts believe that a longer duration of treatment is associated with better outcome (Flores, 2007; Rotgers & Nguyen, 2006). Each session follows a standard structure that allows group members to come away with important information that is relevant to their addiction or other problems in their lives. Even if a person attends only one group, he or she will have been exposed to a model for active, systematic problem solving.

The open-ended nature of the group also means that facilitators must be flexible in implementing session structure. We sometimes encounter cognitive therapists in training who believe that they must cover every component of a cognitive therapy session in a prescribed manner, almost as if they were checking items off of a checklist. In reality, CTAG sessions flow in a smooth, logical manner, and facilitators adapt the structured components on the basis of the group composition (e.g., many new members, one new member, all seasoned members) and the issues that are introduced by group members. We view the key for conducting any cognitive therapy session, including a CTAG session, is that it is driven by strategic consideration of the cognitive model and its application to patients, rather than by a rigid checklist of things that the therapist believes must be covered in the session.

Before providing an overview of the main features of CTAGs, we must acknowledge that many group members have attended or have considered attending other treatment programs and with 12-step programs in particular (e.g., AA, Narcotics Anonymous). In our experience, group members vary substantially in their views and experiences with these programs—some people have had excellent experiences with these programs, whereas others have had negative experiences with the same programs. Many group members have strong, passionate views about 12-step programs (both pro and con). It is important for facilitators to respect all group members' opinions about these experiences and, whenever possible, help group members understand the potential benefits of others' efforts to get help with their addictions. In fact, group members should be encouraged to pursue legitimate treatment services in addition to attending the CTAG, and those who participate in additional treatment can share effective coping strategies that they have learned in other settings.

GOALS OF TREATMENT

As in most addictions treatment approaches, the main goal of CTAGs involves a modification of current and future addictive behavior. However, because treatment takes place in a group format, a second goal of treatment is the fostering of group support and cohesiveness in order to capitalize on this powerful mechanism of change. Facilitators keep both of these goals in mind as they approach any one group session.

Modification of Addictive Behavior

For years there has been controversy regarding the most appropriate goal of addiction treatment—complete abstinence versus controlled use (Miller, 1983). The idea of controlled use can be tied to the concept of *harm reduction* (Des Jarlais, 1995; Roberts & Marlatt, 1999; Karoll, 2010; MacMaster, 2004). Proponents of harm reduction view substance use on a continuum from harm*less* to harm*ful* and believe that even small harm-reducing steps are preferable to no steps. In other words, the harm reduction approach is aimed at decreasing the negative consequences of addictions without insisting upon complete abstinence (Roberts & Marlatt, 1999; Karoll, 2010).

The concept of harm reduction is compatible with cognitive therapy because both emphasize collaboration, empathy, respect, recognition of individual differences, and attention to personal beliefs. With its focus on individualized goal setting, harm reduction is also compatible with the TTM (Prochaska & DiClemente, 2005), discussed in Chapter 3, as it recognizes that not every patient is ready to make substantial changes in his or her life. Moreover, empirical research shows that allowing patients to choose between abstinence and controlled use is associated with better treatment outcome, regardless of the goal that they select (Ojehagen & Berglund, 1989), and that imposing a goal on patients is associated with poorer treatment outcome (Sanchez-Craig & Lei, 1986).

Thus, patients who participate in CTAGs that adopt this philosophy are free to choose whichever goal they believe is best for them—abstinence or controlled use. Both of these goals are respected in these CTAGs, and many patients continue to engage in addictive behavior, at least when they first join the group. Of course, it is also incumbent upon facilitators to work with patients to ensure that their goals are reasonable. For example, there are times when abstinence is indicated, such as when there are specific medical, legal, and/or social consequences associated with continuing to engage in addictive behavior (cf. L. C. Sobell & Sobell, 2011) or when controlled engagement in the addictive behavior would be contraindicated (e.g., smoking). At other times, group members with an alcohol use disorder choose to reduce their drinking to a level that is higher than the recommended limit of no more than three standard drinks on no more than four days per week (M. B. Sobell & Sobell, 1993). In cases in which patients choose goals that would be associated with additional adverse consequences, facilitators can use motivational interviewing (Miller & Rollnick, 2002) to continue to address patients' motivation for change (cf. L. C. Sobell & Sobell, 2011). The key is that goals are developed in a forum that is respectful, nonjudgmental, and open to the possibility that goals will be revisited again in the future.

Although we, ourselves, practice from a harm reduction perspective, we also realize that many addictions counselors operate from an abstinence-only framework. The CTAG can be modified and implemented in an abstinence-only setting. All of the cognitive and behavioral strategies described in this volume can be applied to group members who seek abstinence. The key difference between a CTAG conducted from a harm reduction approach and a CTAG conducted from an abstinence-only approach is that, in the latter, it is assumed that abstinence is the goal of each group member. Psychoeducation provided when patients are oriented to the group (see Chapter 6) is modified to reflect this focus.

The methods for achieving the goal of modifying addictive behavior are twofold. As is stated in Chapter 1, relapse is a common occurrence in people with addictions. In CTAGs, group members are taught to identify cognitive and behavioral determinants of relapse and to develop effective cognitive and behavioral coping strategies that they can use to avoid engaging in addictive behavior. This is the method that is consistent with one that has been used for almost 30 years, the Relapse Prevention approach developed by Marlatt and his colleagues (Larimer, Palmer, & Marlatt, 1999; Marlatt & Donovan, 2005; Marlatt & Witkiewitz , 2005; Witkiewitz & Marlatt, 2004). In the context of the CTAG, relapse prevention is considered in light of the proximal situational cognitive model of addiction, described in Chapter 2, and strategies to modify outcome expectancies and facilitating thoughts, improve coping, and increase self-efficacy are discussed and practiced in session.

A second method for modifying addictive behavior is to address the chronic vulnerabilities that increase the likelihood that group members will have difficulty coping with a trigger. In other words, chronic vulnerabilities are considered in light of the distal background cognitive model of addiction, described in Chapter 2, and strategies to modify unhelpful basic and addiction-related beliefs, manage comorbid psychiatric disorders and unhelpful personality traits, and develop engagement with a healthy support network and in meaningful activities are discussed and practiced in session. Thus, strategies for managing life's challenges and mood disturbance that are not necessarily directly related to the addiction are addressed, with the idea they will reduce stress and build healthy resources on which group members can rely as they overcome their addiction.

Group Cohesiveness and Support

A second goal for CTAGs involves fostering group process itself, as it provides an environment in which powerful change can occur. As Flores (2007) noted, group treatment for patients with addictions is essential because interactions among group members, whether positive or negative, serve as an important vehicle of change. Addictions often leave patients struggling with strife in their interpersonal relationships and shame about aspects of their lives that were adversely affected by their addictive behavior. Fellow group members often provide support that, at times, is more meaningful than support from nonaddicted family members, friends, and even therapists because of their shared experiences. Seasoned group members often provide examples of successes and failures they encountered as they attempted to manage their addictions, which serve as a role model for newer members. What also arises from group cohesiveness, however, are instances when group members hold each other accountable, call each other to task, and provide compelling insights that help each person address his or her denial, commitment to treatment goals, and/or excessive internalization or externalization of his or her problems. Thus, an important job of the facilitator is to recognize these forces and utilize them to promote cognitive and behavioral change.

Monitoring Goals within and across Sessions

On the basis of this framework, within any one session, we encourage facilitators to focus on two aims: (1) the discussion and practice of at least one particular cognitive or behavioral strategy, and (2) the fostering of group cohesiveness and support. In other words, CTAG facilitators strive for a balance between the application and cognitive and behavioral skills to promote change with attention to group process. In our experience, efforts to work on more than these two goals often result in inadequate coverage of any one topic or in the creation of an environment that seems more like a classroom than a psychotherapy group. Facilitators will have a sense of whether they achieved these two aims by the end of group when they seek closure, as group members contemplate the main message that they will take away from the group session.

Facilitators also must be cognizant of balancing emphasis between group and individual goals. Excessive emphasis on group goals runs the risk that the specific needs of individual group members will not be addressed. Conversely, excessive emphasis on individual goals runs the risk that the group will be disjointed, such that it will lack a common thread that connects group members' experiences. Depending on the composition of the group, the facilitator might designate a particular session as a time to review group and individual goals. This exercise would be particularly useful if the majority of the group members have been participating for at least 2 months. However, even group members who have participated for fewer than 2 months can benefit from this discussion, as they will hear firsthand from seasoned group members about the success they have had with applying the cognitive and behavioral strategies in their daily lives and with maintaining either abstinence or controlled engagement in their addictive behavior. Thus, a periodic review of progress toward goals can instill hope in newer group members.

It is also important to periodically monitor goals across sessions because they might change throughout the course of treatment. Some group members might enroll in the CTAG when they are in an earlier stage of change (e.g., precontemplation, contemplation), and after seeing some positive changes in their lives and hearing testimonials from other group members, they move into the preparation or action stage. We have also seen group members begin treatment with a goal consistent with the harm reduction approach, only to modify their goals to focus on abstinence after continued participation in the group. When facilitators periodically review treatment goals and identify this transition, they can mobilize the group member's motivation to make concrete changes in his or her life.

CTAG PARTICIPANTS

Facilitators

CTAG facilitators are mental health professionals trained to conduct group cognitive therapy. These professionals may be psychologists, psychiatrists, social workers, certified drug and alcohol counselors, psychiatric nurses, or certified counselors. It is essential that facilitators have a working knowledge of the nature of addictive behavior, the cognitive model of addictions, and the cognitive and behavioral strategies for managing addictions that are described in Part II. Facilitators should also be able to conceptualize group members' clinical presentations quickly and accurately and must, therefore, have a working knowledge of psychopathology (i.e., DSM-IV-TR; American Psychiatric Association, 2000).

According to White (2000), there are several characteristics of successful facilitators of a cognitive therapy group: (1) the ability to promote and model active participation, (2) the ability to create an environment that promotes an openness to individual differences, (3) the effective use of collaboration with group members and Socratic questioning, and (4) the use of "we" language to communicate a universality of shared experiences. In addition, CTAG facilitators need strong interpersonal skills, such as warmth, genuineness, spontaneity, attentiveness, and empathy. Facilitating a group can be stimulating and rewarding at times, and stressful or even boring at other times. The challenge for the facilitator is to respond to the mood of the group in a way that furthers, rather than hinders, its progress.

It is optimal to have two co-facilitators in order to monitor reactions of each group member and present different perspectives on and examples of cognitive and behavioral coping strategies. For example, one facilitator can monitor group process and identify opportunities to incorporate group participation while the other facilitator is providing psychoeducation (cf. Monti et al., 2002). In many instances, one co-facilitator will be an experienced clinician who has run the group for some time, whereas the other co-facilitator will be a trainee who is getting supervised experience to specialize in treatment for addictions populations. Co-facilitators typically meet before each group in order to clarify roles, prepare new material, and address any issues pertaining to individual group members or group process. They also debrief after the session has been completed so that they can evaluate the degree to which the application of cognitive and behavioral strategies was successful and plan for any corrective action that might be necessary in the subsequent session (Bieling et al., 2006).

One specific issue that often arises when developing treatments for addictive disorders is whether it is required that the facilitator has a personal history of addiction. It is our stance that a personal history of addictive behavior is not a requirement to facilitate CTAGs and that it is the personal choice of each facilitator to decide whether or not to disclose such information. However, if a facilitator is actively engaging in addictive behavior to a degree that it interferes with his or her ability to successfully treat these (and other) patients, then it is recommended that he or she discontinue his or her role as facilitator until the addiction has been treated.

Group Members

CTAGs consist of between 5 and 12 group members. This broad range might strike many readers as odd. However, it reflects the reality faced by facilitators who implement CTAGs in diverse settings. Because of its open format, facilitators might not always have a sense of the number of group members who will attend in any one session. Some days, all patients who have been recruited for the group might be in attendance; on other days, only a few patients might be in attendance. In fact, we have even held CTAGs with fewer than 5 members when fewer than 5 members have shown up! In general, we find that having at least 5 members in attendance helps the group to be interactive and stimulating; groups often become disjointed and difficult to follow with more than 12 members (cf. Bieling et al., 2006). Research also shows that group cohesiveness is optimal when there are between 5 and 9 members (Burlingame et al., 2001) Thus, we encourage facilitators to aim for a group of 5 to 9 members, to cap off group membership with 12 members, but also to recognize that there might be special circumstances that require an additional 1 or 2 members to be enrolled.

Contrary to stereotypes, people with addictive disorders comprise a heterogeneous group. They differ in the substances they use, in their patterns of use, and in their personalities. Some will be lonely and depressed with limited resources, whereas others might be financially secure, with meaningful relationships and satisfying careers. Some, but not all, will have significant mental health problems. We view this heterogeneity as an asset to CTAGs, as the wide range of struggles can be conceptualized from a cognitive behavioral perspective, and members will be exposed to a diverse array of situations and circumstances in which cognitive and behavioral strategies can be applied.

Although the philosophy that underlies the CTAG is that heterogeneity is a strength of this treatment approach, there are characteristics of some potential patients that raise "red flags" regarding their ability to be an active and supportive group member. For example, florid positive symptoms or prominent negative symptoms of a psychotic disorder might preclude a potential group member from acquiring the coping skills that are discussed in session. In addition, florid positive symptoms of a psychotic disorder or behaviors associated with some personality disorders might disrupt the presentation of information in session and meaningful interactions among group members. Some CTAG members might have significant psychiatric, medical, or vocational problems that require even more immediate attention than their addiction.

However, we would caution facilitators against ruling out a potential group member on the basis of a psychiatric diagnosis alone. As is discussed in the next section, the presence of one or more psychiatric diagnoses must be considered in conjunction with a potential group member's suitability for cognitive therapy, interpersonal skill, and primary presenting problem before making a final determination of inclusion into the CTAG. Moreover, potential group members who are struggling with a variety of issues are strongly encouraged to receive the appropriate treatment and other services in addition to their participation in the CTAG. Our rule of thumb is that if potential group members have the capacity to understand the content that is discussed in group and interact appropriately with the facilitators and other group members, and they are addressing other issues or problems that have the potential to affect their group participation in other treatment settings, then they are likely to be good candidates for the CTAG.

PREPARATION FOR GROUP PARTICIPATION

Prior to enrolling a person into the CTAG, it is important to have an individual meeting with him or her in order to understand the nature of his or her addiction and readiness for change, conduct a psychological assessment, determine his or her suitability for a group cognitive therapy approach, educate about the nature of the group and its rules, and set individual goals (see Figure 4.2). During this interview, the facilitators can begin to gather information about the distal background and proximal situational factors associated with the person's addictive behavior, which will allow them to begin formulating a cognitive case conceptualization (see Chapter 5).

The most obvious activity that occurs in the context of an individual meeting with a potential group member is discussion of the frequency, severity, and longevity of his or her addictive disorder and the degree to which he or she is ready for change. On the one hand, facilitators ensure that the addictive behavior is problematic enough to be considered an addictive disorder, as that will be the focus of the group and the problem reported by all of the other group members. On the other hand, facilitators also must

---

- Understand the nature of the potential group member's addiction and readiness for change.
- Conduct a psychological assessment.
- Determine the potential group member's suitability for the cognitive therapy approach.
- Educate about the nature of the group and its rules.
- Set individual goals.

FIGURE 4.2. Goals of the pregroup interview.

determine whether a higher level of care is indicated before participation in the CTAG, such as detoxification. Potential group members who need a higher level of care are often referred for such treatment, with the understanding that they will eventually participate in the CTAG when they are ready to do so. Facilitators also assess for the presence of polydrug abuse or other co-occurring addiction problems that might also be the focus of this person's group treatment. A straightforward approach to assessing readiness for change is to ask the potential group member, "Would you say that you are not ready to change in the next 6 months [corresponds to precontemplation], are thinking about changing in the next 6 months [corresponds to contemplation], are thinking about changing in the next month [corresponds to preparation], or have already made some progress [corresponds to action]?" (Norcross et al., 2011).

The psychological assessment includes diagnostic interview questions that identify the presence or absence of major Axis I and Axis II disorders, including depression, bipolar disorder, anxiety disorders, psychotic disorders, and personality disorders. As has been stated up to this point in this volume, many symptoms of these disorders are common in patients with addictions and are addressed at certain times in the CTAG, such as depression, anxiety, and relationship problems. However, the CTAG should not be viewed as a substitute for the treatment of these disorders. The most severe symptoms of some of these disorders, such as suicidal behavior, nonsuicidal self-injury behavior, or rapid cycling, are not addressed in the CTAG and always require immediate attention by a professional outside the group context. Potential group members with any psychiatric disorder should be referred for services such as individual psychotherapy or medication management, with the recommendation that they should be receiving these treatments concurrently with their participation in the CTAG. In the case of potential group members with moderate to severe symptoms of one or more psychiatric disorder, facilitators have the discretion to make participation in other treatments a requirement.

Making determinations of the severity of a person's addictive disorder and associated psychiatric symptoms can be made using diagnostic interviews such as the Structured Clinical Interview for DSM-IV-TR Axis I Disorders (SCID-I/P; First, Spitzer, Gibbon, & Williams, 2002) or the Addiction Severity Index (ASI; McLellan et al., 1985). These interviews offer clear criteria for determining whether a person meets criteria for an addictive or psychiatric disorder. In contrast, many clinicians find it more difficult to determine whether a potential group member is suitable for the cognitive therapy approach. In their now classic book, Safran and Segal (1990) outlined many characteristics that make a person especially well suited to cognitive therapy, such as the ability to identify cognitions, the ability to identify associated emotions and differentiate among a number of emotional states, a sense of personal responsibility for change, the degree to which his or her presenting problem can be understood in light of the cognitive model, the ability to focus on a specific problem, the ability to form a strong therapeutic alliance, and optimism about treatment. Facilitators can use the interview included in Safran and Segal's appendix I, or at least can keep these principles in mind as they conduct the interview with the potential group member. If the potential group member does not buy into the cognitive therapy approach, or if he or she demonstrates an interpersonal style that has the potential to create difficulties in forming relationships with the facilitators or other group members, then it is possible that the CTAG might not be an appropriate outlet for treatment.

That being said, we realize that there are many settings in which there are limited options for treatment of certain problems, such as addictions. We have heard from many clinicians that, in their facilities, the choice is to enroll a patient in a CTAG or nothing. Thus, some clinicians might find themselves in a position in which they feel pulled to enroll a person in the CTAG despite the fact that the cognitive approach does not seem well suited to conceptualizing his or her addictive behaviors, or the fact that he or she exhibited some concerning interpersonal behaviors during the pre-group interview. We have seen many instances in which a person deemed not to be well suited for a CTAG nevertheless benefited greatly. To achieve a positive outcome with these patients, we encourage facilitators to (1) regard participation in the first few sessions as a "trial" period and, thereafter, evaluate the degree to which the patient's participation is working out for all involved; (2) use creative approaches to illustrate the manner in which the comprehensive cognitive model of addiction is applicable to them; (3) reinforce cognitive and behavior changes, even if they seem minor; (4) regularly check in with them to monitor understanding and progress; and (5) set firm limits and boundaries regarding any disruptive behavior.

During the consideration of their suitability for the CTAG, potential group members will be educated about the nature of the group and what they can expect will happen in session. Facilitators educate potential group members about the comprehensive cognitive model of addiction, identify aspects of the model that particularly resonate with these patients, and demonstrate the manner in which coping strategies emerge from the application of this model. They also describe the types of activities that take place in the group setting, including the expectation that each group member will give a brief introduction, that cognitive and behavioral strategies will be discussed and often practiced in the session, and the expectation that group members will engage in between-session work (i.e., homework) in order to generalize the strategies that are discussed and practiced in session to their daily lives. Facilitators can share common topics that are often discussed in group and the types of problems that are often endorsed by group members. Furthermore, they discuss their stance on abstinence versus harm reduction and the participation in other treatment programs. As facilitators are providing this information, they regularly check in and obtain feedback to ensure that the potential group member understands what is being presented and believes that this approach would be helpful.

In addition to education about the cognitive model and general approach to therapy, facilitators also specify the group rules. In fact, it is wise to have the group rules written down on a sheet of paper, with a space at the bottom where the potential group member can place his or her signature, to ensure that adequate time has been allocated to discussion of group rules and that the potential group member agrees to them (cf. Bernard et al., 2008). Then, the agreement can be placed in the patient's chart, and the patient can take a signed copy of the group rules home with him or her. Facilitators can develop whatever group rules they believe are necessary on the basis of their clinical experience and rules of their facility. Two fundamental group rules that are covered in every CTAG are (1) the notion of confidentiality, such that group members must agree not to divulge identifying information about another group member outside of the session; and (2) the expectation that group members will not be under the influence of alcohol or drugs at the time of the session (cf. Monti et al., 2002; L. C. Sobell & Sobell, 2011). Other basic rules that we have found to be important are (1) treating others with consideration and respect; (2) talking honestly and personally about themselves, rather than philosophizing, generalizing, distancing, or talking about others; and (3) turning off cell phones during session. Not only does such a discussion of group rules set clear expectations for each member's role in the group, it also provides a basis for remediation and possible dismissal from the group in the future if the group member repeatedly violates these rules.

Finally, we encourage facilitators to work with new group members to specify their individual goals for the CTAG. The reader has seen that some group members have vague goals for decreasing addictive behavior but have not yet implemented a plan of action for doing so, that some express an overt wish to cut down on their substance use, that some may wish to become completely abstinent, and that some may have been abstinent for some time and desire group membership for its supportive quality. The goals of each individual member are respected, provided that they are consistent with the general criteria discussed in this chapter and the philosophy of the treatment program, and facilitators apply cognitive and behavioral strategies to help them develop tools to achieve these goals. Individual group members also might formulate additional goals, such as reducing depression, improving relationships with others, or making other positive changes in their lives.

STRUCTURE OF THE CTAG

Each CTAG session follows a standard structure that can be adapted in a flexible manner, depending on the composition of the group at any one session. Such a structure allows new group members to assimilate rather quickly into the group process. In addition, adherence to the structure ensures that each group member has an opportunity to participate actively, that the cognitive model of addictions is presented and applied to group members' concerns, and that by the end of the session, group members will have been exposed to at least one tangible strategy to manage their addictions, associated mood problems, or other issues. Each session consists of the following components:

1. *Facilitator introductions.* Facilitators introduce themselves, the group rules, and the basic features of the cognitive approach.
2. *Group member introductions.* Group members introduce themselves, and the facilitators begin to relate their problems to the cognitive model.
3. *Cognitive and behavioral strategy(ies).* Group members might develop strategies to identify and evaluate thoughts and beliefs that lead them to engage in addictive behaviors or that exacerbate other problems in their lives. They also might be taught specific coping skills relevant to their current problems (e.g., urges and cravings, repairing close relationships, mood disturbance, unhealthy lifestyle). The specific strategy or strategies selected are dependent upon the issues group members discussed during introductions, as well as material that had been discussed in the previous session.
5. *Homework.* Each group member has the opportunity to review his or her between-session work and commits to new between-session work in order to achieve his or her goals.
6. *Closure.* Members reflect on what they have learned in the group session.

Facilitator and Group Member Introductions

At each CTAG session, facilitators introduce themselves, and then group members introduce themselves with their (1) names, (2) addictions (past and present), (3) status of their addictions (last use, urges, cravings), (4) goals for change, and (5) other issues (e.g., interpersonal problems, anger control, legal problems). During these introductions, facilitators keep group members focused, offer encouragement, and bridge from previous sessions. They also highlight common themes among group members. Often these themes emerge from the "other issues" section of members' introductions. The common theme can then become the focus for the session after members have introduced themselves. At an appropriate time during member introductions, facilitators introduce and review the cognitive model of addictions by applying it directly to group members having the most difficulty or success in their recovery.

Cognitive and Behavioral Strategies

This segment of the group session is the "heart" of the CTAG, as it is at this point in the session that cognitive and behavioral approaches for managing addictive behavior and other issues are presented, discussed, and practiced (cf. Rotgers & Nguyen, 2006). Facilitators can be flexible and collaborative in deciding upon a specific focus for the application of cognitive and behavioral strategies. For example, facilitators might detect a sense of urgency in the concerns expressed by several group members and identify a particular coping skill that would address the pressing concerns brought up in the introductions. In contrast, facilitators might be working actively across several sessions to reinforce the acquisition of cognitive restructuring skills (see Chapter 7), and it would be logical to continue this work in the current session, reinforcing group members' completion of homework and applying the skills to the concerns identified in the introductions.

In Part II, we have included separate chapters to describe cognitive strategies (i.e., those that are used to evaluate unhelpful thoughts and beliefs) and other cognitive and behavioral coping strategies. However, it is important for facilitators to keep in mind that the distinction between cognitive and behavioral strategies is often arbitrary, and, most often, the evaluation of thoughts and beliefs and the development of coping skills occur *simultaneously.* Thus, it is quite common for a facilitator to recognize a theme in group members' reported difficulties and then address the theme using *both* cognitive strategies and behavioral coping skills strategies. For example, if facilitators recognize that the group would benefit by focusing on repairing close relationships, then they might identify thoughts and beliefs that interfere with repairing close relationships *as well as* concrete skills for managing and improving these relationships. If facilitators see that several members are struggling with urges and cravings, then they might decide to focus on cognitive strategies to evaluate facilitating thoughts and develop control beliefs *as well as* on other cognitive and behavioral skills for coping with cravings. If facilitators sense that a number of members are experiencing concurrent symptoms of depression and anxiety, then they might use cognitive strategies to evaluate depressive and anxious thoughts *as well as* behavioral strategies for improving mood, such as activity scheduling or muscle relaxation. The format of CTAGs allows for facilitators to use clinical judgment and creativity in conceptualizing group members' needs from a cognitive behavioral perspective and select appropriate cognitive and coping skills interventions on the basis of that conceptualization.

Homework

Homework assignments are designed to help patients achieve the goals they set in treatment. At times, facilitators identify instances for group members to recommit themselves to their goals and to decide on one specific way they will move toward their goals in the time between sessions. Other homework assignments involve group members practicing the cognitive and behavioral strategies discussed or practiced in session so that they can generalize these skills to their daily lives. Regardless of the specific nature of the homework assignment, facilitators consistently emphasize its importance for success in participation in CTAGs. Research shows that there is a strong association between success in individual therapy and homework compliance (Addis & Jacobson, 2000), and we expect that the same association would hold true for participation in group cognitive therapy.

Of course, when homework is developed and committed to by group members, it is imperative that the facilitators revisit the assignment in the subsequent session (Rotgers & Nguyen, 2006). Not doing so runs the risk of communicating to group members that homework is not important. Discussion of the manner in which group members implemented homework allows group members to revel in their successes and receive feedback from others when they encounter difficulties. Discussion of the previous week's homework assignment can take place at several points in a CTAG session, such as during introductions or during the portion of group focused on developing cognitive or behavioral skills. Some expert cognitive therapists even recommend having group members turn in written homework to facilitators at the beginning of the session, which increases accountability (Bieling et al., 2006).

Closure

The final minutes of group are reserved for closure. Closure is imperative for group members to solidify the information they learned during that group session, verbalize any reactions to the discussions that ensued in the group, and make a commitment to implement the homework assignment. It is an opportunity for group members to articulate the most important message they are taking away from the session (cf. L. C. Sobell & Sobell, 2011). Closure allows for facilitators to develop a sense of whether group members understood the material being presented and have the potential to apply it to their lives. If it is clear that group members indeed understood the material and have a plan for practicing the strategy, then facilitators note this so the strategy can be taught again in future CTAG sessions and so that they can continue to reinforce its use in returning members. If it seems that group members have not understood the material or anticipate difficulty using it in their lives, then facilitators take care to identify obstacles that might have interfered with the learning of this material and ways to overcome those obstacles.

OVERVIEW OF THIS MANUAL

The remainder of this manual provides a guide for conducting CTAGs. In the following chapters, strategies and procedures for conducting each component of a CTAG session are described, including introductions, evaluation of thoughts and beliefs, acquisition of coping skills, and homework and closure. In addition, we have devoted a chapter to the process of cognitive case conceptualization, which will help facilitators apply the comprehensive cognitive model of addiction, theory associated with group process, and the TTM to individual group members and to the group as a whole. Readers are encouraged to read the entire manual prior to conducting their first CTAG and then consult the manual selectively as groups get underway in order to address specific issues and difficulties. Case vignettes are presented to illustrate the application of CTAG structure and strategy.

CHAPTER 5 | Cognitive Case Conceptualization

The cognitive case conceptualization is an understanding of a person's clinical presentation in the context of the comprehensive cognitive model of addiction, described in Chapter 2. That is, it is a process by which cognitive therapists apply cognitive theory to the individual patient. It incorporates a number of cognitive, emotional, behavioral, and social or environmental factors that are relevant to understanding the person's clinical presentation—both his or her addictive behavior, as well as comorbid psychiatric symptoms. This information provides an in-depth understanding of the manner in which group members developed addictions and helps to answer many questions about their life experiences and basic beliefs, which in turn sheds light on the manner in which they respond to slips, stressors, failure, and disappointment. It also illustrates the cognitive, behavioral, and emotional sequence of events that occurs when people are faced with a trigger to engage in addictive behavior and the factors that increase or decrease the likelihood that they will have a lapse or relapse.

The cognitive case conceptualization is developed and revised over time. Facilitators begin to formulate the conceptualization after they have met individually with the potential group member. However, the level of detail that they obtain from that meeting usually only allows them to develop hypotheses about that person's distal background and proximal situational factors that underlie his or her addictive behavior. As more information is collected from the person's participation in group sessions, facilitators expand the conceptualization, verifying hypotheses that were initially generated or developing more refined hypotheses. This understanding then guides facilitators in developing strategic interventions that are most likely to be helpful in reducing the likelihood of relapse and decreasing associated psychiatric symptoms. Thus, the cognitive case conceptualization is a work in progress that develops throughout the course of treatment.

There are two cognitive case conceptualizations that facilitators must develop—that of each individual group member, and that of the group as a whole. As is seen throughout this chapter, there are strategic questions that facilitators can ask at opportune moments to probe about group members' early experiences, basic beliefs, addiction-related beliefs, triggers, outcome expectancies, and facilitating thoughts. In the remainder of this chapter, we describe the manner in which cognitive case conceptualizations can be developed for the group and its members presented in Chapter 1.

FORMULATING THE COGNITIVE CASE CONCEPTUALIZATION OF THE INDIVIDUAL CLINICAL PRESENTATION

Cognitive case conceptualizations of individual group members' clinical presentations serve many purposes. First, they help facilitators to sort through a great deal of information in a systematic way on the basis of cognitive theory. This process allows facilitators to gain clarity as they identify the cognitive, behavioral, emotional, and social or environmental factors that maintain a group member's addictive behavior. Because CTAGs are open groups, meaning that group members can come and go as they please, some group members' attendance may be sporadic. The cognitive case conceptualization helps facilitators to quickly review the primary psychological factors associated with those group members' addictive behavior so that they can continue to move forward with those individuals, rather than taking a step backward and reviewing their background information and presenting problems in excessive detail. The cognitive case conceptualization, then, serves as a template to quickly assimilate new information and compare it with information that has already been obtained in previous sessions. Second, development of the cognitive case conceptualization capitalizes on two important processes of change specified in the TTM (Prochaska & DiClemente, 2005)—consciousness raising, such that group members learn more about the interplay of cognitive, behavioral, emotional, and social or environmental factors that underlie their addiction, and self-reevaluation, in which they assess their specific thoughts and feelings about themselves. Group members may even experience dramatic relief as they attend to aspects of their conceptualizations and as they express affect about their life problems.

Figure 5.1 summarizes the information that facilitators typically consider in formulating an individual cognitive case conceptualization. Two realms of information contribute to the cognitive case conceptualization of patients with addictions: (1) a *distal background profile*, and (2) a *proximal*

DISTAL BACKGROUND FACTORS

- Family history of addiction and psychiatric disorders
- Relevant personality traits
- Current and past psychiatric disorders
- Early life experiences with family, peers, and success/failure
- Exposure to and experimentation with addictive behavior
- Social support network
- Engagement in meaningful activities
- Basic beliefs
- Addiction-related beliefs

PROXIMAL SITUATIONAL FACTORS

- Anticipatory outcome expectancies
- Relief-oriented outcome expectancies
- Facilitating thoughts
- Urges and cravings
- Self-efficacy
- Repertoire of coping behaviors
- Attentional biases toward addiction-related stimuli

FIGURE 5.1. Information included in the individual cognitive case conceptualization.

situational profile. The distal background profile is composed of the information in the distal background cognitive model of addiction, described in Chapter 2 (i.e., Figure 2.5). This information includes a group member's genetic vulnerability, personality traits, psychiatric diagnoses, early experiences, and current environment that make him or her vulnerable to engage in continued addictive behavior. The proximal situational profile is composed of the information in the proximal situational cognitive model of addiction, described in Chapter 2 (i.e., Figure 2.3). This information includes triggers, addiction-related outcome expectancies, facilitating thoughts, urges and cravings, self-efficacy, coping strategies, and attentional biases toward addiction-relevant stimuli. Together, these sources of information help facilitators to understand the factors that made group members vulnerable to develop addictions, the beliefs about addictions that serve as reinforcers, triggers that provide a context for engagement in the addictive behavior in particular situations, and the sequence of cognitions that exacerbate urges and cravings and that eventually result in a slip or a lapse. In the subsequent sections, we illustrate strategies for gathering these two realms of information.

Distal Background Profile

Construction of the distal background profile involves collecting information about group members' family history, past experiences (e.g., family, social, economic, exposure to addictive behavior), current environment, psychiatric diagnoses, and personality traits, and considering the manner in which these factors shed light on their current clinical presentation. As facilitators generate a distal background profile, they develop hypotheses about group members' basic beliefs that developed over time about themselves (e.g., "I'm worthless"), the world (e.g., "The world is cruel"), or the future (e.g., "Things will never get better"). Some ideas for phrasing questions that speak to these basic beliefs include "What messages have you received from others about yourself? About the way the world works? About what's in store for the future?" For example, if a group member believes that he or she cannot cope with problems without using alcohol, the facilitator might ask, "As a child, what messages did you receive about your competency and ability to cope?" In addition, facilitators ask specific questions to identify beliefs that fueled the development of addictive behavior, such as the anticipation of positive outcomes (e.g., fitting in with the crowd) or relief from negative outcomes (e.g., avoiding anxiety). Figure 5.2 summarizes questions to elicit information that is often included in the distal background profile. The following vignette illustrates the manner in which facilitators elicit information to refine distal background profiles for several group members. The construction of the distal background profile starts with Michael's comment that he is judgmental of himself:

> MICHAEL: I'm judgmental of myself. I always think I should achieve more and be more like other people rather than myself.
>
> FACILITATOR 1: From where did you learn that?
>
> MICHAEL: I guess going back to my childhood; my parents gave me signals to be like my older brother.
>
> FACILITATOR 2: Do you remember any specifics about that?
>
> MICHAEL: Yeah, my dad and my brother were both handymen, always working in the garage. I liked to do things that were indoors, you know, like work on the computer.
>
> FACILITATOR 2: How did that affect your relationship with your father?

- Did anyone in your family have a problem with addictions? If so, what was it like growing up with that person? What role did that addiction play in your family?
- How did your family generally cope with stress or adversity?
- What messages did you receive about your competency or ability to cope effectively?
- What messages did you receive about your worth as a human being?
- What messages did you receive about your ability to achieve goals?
- What was your peer group like when you were a child? What messages did you get about yourself and the world from your peer interactions?
- When you first started to engage in addictive behavior, what did it teach you about yourself and the world? Did the addiction somehow make life easier for you to handle?
- What aspects of your personality do you believe make you vulnerable to addiction? In what ways have these personality traits caused problems for you?
- Have you ever been diagnosed with a psychiatric disorder? If so, what role do you think that plays in your addiction?
- Who do you view as being there to provide support to you? Are you satisfied with the size of this support network? Are you satisfied with the frequency of interactions with people in this support network? Are there times when you view the support that these people provide as unhelpful?
- How do you spend your time when you are not engaging in addictive behavior? Do you view these activities as meaningful or fulfilling?

FIGURE 5.2. Sample questions to identify distal background factors.

MICHAEL: It wasn't good. He thought "real men's" work was working with your hands and being outdoors, not being an intellectual and working on the computer.

FACILITATOR 1: I'm sensing that your relationship with your father was distant, and that your brother had a stronger relationship with your father.

MICHAEL: Yeah, that's exactly it. And my mom used to bug me to spend more time with my dad and brother, but I just couldn't bring myself to do it. It just seemed like I was such an outsider. And it wasn't like they were making the effort to invite me to spend time with them.

FACILITATOR 2: What sorts of messages did you get from this situation?

MICHAEL: I guess all of this led to low self-esteem. That I was somehow a lesser person than them. That there was something wrong with me because I didn't like things that men should like.

FACILITATOR 1: How did sex get in the picture? Were you exposed to sex or pornography at an early age?

MICHAEL: Like a lot of guys, when I was a teenager I found my father's magazines and would steal them from time to time.

FACILITATOR 1: Do you remember your first experience looking at your dad's magazines?

MICHAEL: Oh yeah.

FACILITATOR 1: What ran through your mind during that experience?

MICHAEL: It sounds stupid to say this aloud, but my thought was that I'm finally a man.

FACILITATOR 1: And how did you feel then?

MICHAEL: I felt better, finally somewhat happy because I felt that I was a competent male. Now that I think about it, since the magazines were my father's, I guess I thought that I was doing something that he would approve of.

FACILITATOR 1: (*turning to the group*) What we've done here is identify some important components of the distal background profile that underlies Michael's sex addiction. This means that we've helped to identify some of his early experiences, basic beliefs about himself, and beliefs about sex or pornography that have contributed to and reinforced his addiction. An early experience that is particularly relevant to Michael's addiction is that he perceived that he was excluded from the relationship between his father and brother, and he sensed that his father did not respect things Michael was good at. This probably contributed to Michael's basic belief that he is incompetent, particularly incompetent as a man. But when he started to look at his father's magazines, he got the sense that he was finally accepted by someone "manly" like his father. So he developed a powerful addiction-related belief—"I'm now competent as a man"—when he viewed pornography. Michael, would you say that this belief generalized to other behaviors that were related to looking at your father's magazines, like having casual sexual relationships?

MICHAEL: Most definitely. It was like every time I had sex with someone the other guys wanted, I was more and more powerful. I think I was addicted to that power.

Discussions such as this can be invaluable in providing information for facilitators to develop and refine cognitive case conceptualizations of individual group members' clinical presentations, as well as to reinforce the components of the cognitive model to group members. However, it is important for facilitators to balance the targeted cognitive behavioral focus on any one group member with attention to group dynamics as a whole. Falling into the trap of essentially doing individual therapy with any one person in the group context runs the risk of failing to mobilize group interactions and support as a mechanism of change that is just as important as the acquisition of cognitive and behavioral strategies to manage addictive behavior (Flores, 2007; Yalom & Leszcz, 2005). Thus, facilitators are mindful of the principles of universality, in which they help group members to see that there are many similarities in their struggles, and group cohesiveness. The following is a vignette that illustrates the manner in which the facilitators brought support and insight from other group members as they began to develop a distal background profile with Dave, after Dave made a comment suggesting that he did not view the discussion as particularly useful:

DAVE: I don't get why all of this is important.

FACILITATOR 1: I'm glad you said that, Dave. We want to be sure that everyone understands this model and the way it applies to their own addiction. If we can figure out the basic beliefs and addiction-related beliefs that keep our addiction going, then we'll be able to use this group to figure out ways to modify those beliefs, and ultimately decrease the likelihood of a slip or a relapse. In Michael's case, he's been developing skills for modifying the idea that he is incompetent. I wonder if we can develop a distal background profile with you, Dave, so that its relevance might be more apparent to you. Maybe some of the group members who have been participating in the CTAG for a longer period of time can help you? (*Michael, Ellen, and Brian nod.*)

DAVE: (*looking skeptical*) I'm not sure what you want to know. My father drank and smoked weed. My mother drank. All of my friends drank, did drugs, and got in a lot of trouble. That's the environment I grew up in.

FACILITATOR 1: All very important pieces of information, Dave. You were exposed to alcohol and drug use early, as a way of life. Does anyone have an idea about why that piece of information is so important?

BRIAN: 'Cause that was all he knew.

ELLEN: Yes, I agree with Brian. It makes a lot of sense that you're having drinking problems now, if that's what you saw day in and day out when you were growing up.

DAVE: (*slight nod of head*)

FACILITATOR 1: Often when we are exposed to alcohol, drugs, or other addictions at an early age, we develop strong beliefs about the role they play in our lives. What messages did you get about alcohol and drugs?

DAVE: (*slightly irritated*) I don't know.

FACILITATOR 1: Remember what we just found out about Michael—that he got the message that looking at pornography and having casual sexual relationships made him more of a man. It is logical that a belief like that would fuel his sex addiction. Does anyone have any ideas about beliefs that would develop from early exposure to alcohol and drug use?

ALLISON: My uncle is an alcoholic, and my cousins grew up in an alcoholic household. Now that they're adults, three out of the four of them are alcoholics themselves. I think they learned that drinking was a way to escape their problems. I don't know if that's helpful to you or not, Dave.

DAVE: There were *always* problems. Dad never paid the bills on time. My sister got pregnant when she was 15. And then I got kicked out of school after I started a fight with one of the teachers.

MICHAEL: Do you think alcohol and drug use in your home growing up contribute to these problems?

DAVE: (*pausing slightly*) I guess so. My dad was dead to the world half the time, so he never knew if I was coming or going. And we couldn't live in a better place because they weren't responsible with money.

FACILITATOR 2: So what did you learn about drinking and doing drugs from that?

DAVE: (*sighing*) I guess that it is more fun to have a drink or take a hit than deal with our miserable lives. Yeah, now that I think about it, drinking or doing drugs was the only time I saw my dad happy. At least happy until he got so drunk that he passed out. The problems went away, at least for a little bit.

FACILITATOR 1: You've identified two important addiction-related beliefs—that drinking and doing drugs are the only way to have fun, and that they help problems go away. Would you say that you have adopted your father's beliefs?

DAVE: I don't know, I would like to think I have more going for me than my father.

ELLEN: It certainly seems like you have one very important thing going for you—that you've come here to get help. I, for one, am glad that you're here. (*Other group members nod their heads.*)

FACILITATOR 1: I agree wholeheartedly. (*Facilitator 2 nods vigorously.*) I'll regard these two beliefs as hypotheses, or guesses about the beliefs that underlie your drinking and drug use, and as we get to know one another better, I'll check back with you to see if they're accurate. Is that OK with you?

DAVE: OK.

Notice in this example that Dave was not ready to acknowledge his addiction-related beliefs, so Facilitator 1 took care not to impose them on him and instead regarded them as working hypotheses. As Dave attends more groups, the facilitators will continue to gather information about his history, which may or may not support the original conceptualization of his beliefs, and will modify their hypotheses as necessary.

The distal background profile identifies basic beliefs and addiction-related beliefs that contribute not only to addictive behaviors, but also to other psychiatric problems. Over the course of the first few group sessions in which Dave participated, the facilitators developed the hypothesis that Dave has two basic beliefs: "I need to look out for myself" and "No one cares." These beliefs, in combination with the demeanor in which he presents himself in group, raise the possibility that Dave is characterized by some features of antisocial personality disorder (ASPD). In other words, Dave presents as a person who is "out for himself" and rarely considers the impact of his behavior on others. His behavior confirms this impression, as he has had trouble with the law, has been fired from several jobs, and has a history of getting in physical altercations. As is seen in the subsequent vignette, Ellen also has the basic belief, "No one cares." However, this belief is not associated with a clinical presentation consistent with ASPD; rather, this belief, along with a belief that she is unlovable, supports the impression that she is depressed. It turned out that some other group members resonated with her experience:

FACILITATOR 1: We've identified some very powerful beliefs in Michael and Dave that influence their addictive behavior, and more generally, the manner in which they approach challenges in their lives. Ellen, I'd like to turn back to you, since we identified earlier that you struggle with depression in addition to an overeating addiction. How might these problems be related to messages you received while you were growing up?

ELLEN: I'm not sure. I've never been that thin, and to some degree, I have always turned to sweets as comfort food when I am down or upset about something. But the eating really became a problem after my divorce.

BRIAN: What was it about the divorce that made you start eating so much?

ELLEN: (*becoming tearful again*) I just felt so lost, so alone. When I was younger, I never thought I would ever get married. And even though my marriage wasn't great, it was better than being alone.

MICHAEL: You never thought you would get married? Why is that?

ELLEN: I don't know, I was just so shy, so "blah" as a child. I have seven brothers and sisters, and it seemed like one of them was always in the spotlight. People seemed to forget that I existed.

FACILITATOR 1: And what did that mean to you?

ELLEN: That I was invisible, that no one cared.

FACILITATOR 1: Interestingly, you have a similar basic belief as Dave— that no one cared. He also has the belief that he should just take care of himself. Did you develop that idea as well?

ELLEN: No, I think I was the opposite. I didn't have the confidence that I could take care of myself. So I just crawled back into my shell.

FACILITATOR 2: Would you say that you struggled with depression even when you were a child?

ELLEN: Oh yes, I'm sure of it.

FACILITATOR 2: And do you think that might have been related to your belief that no one cared?

ELLEN: Yes, absolutely. I felt like no one loved me, not even my own parents.

FACILITATOR 1: You have the basic beliefs that no one cares and no one loves you. Now let's fast forward to the divorce. How did these beliefs translate into a problem with overeating?

ELLEN: Because I was so low at that point, food was like my only friend. My children were teenagers then, and they decided to live with my husband. I had nothing. Food was the only thing that gave me any bit of enjoyment.

FACILITATOR 1: I'm sorry to hear all of this, Ellen. That sounds like a very difficult time for you. Do you think some of these beliefs are still operating now?

ELLEN: Yes, I suppose they are. I guess that's why I'm here.

ALLISON: Wow, I can really relate to all of this.

FACILITATOR 2: In what way, Allison?

ALLISON: Well, before I started in this group, I just assumed that I smoked because everyone around me smoked. That's what it's like when you grow up on the reservation.

FACILITATOR 2: It sounds like our discussion has given you some new insights. What might those new insights be?

ALLISON: I kind of had the belief that others didn't care as well. But it was also a little bit different in my case. My mom paid a lot of attention to me, at least in her own way when she was around. It was the other kids at school who didn't.

FACILITATOR 2: And what did that tell you about yourself?

ALLISON: That I wasn't good enough. I especially felt like that when I moved off the reservation and switched schools. There were a lot of girls who were from families that had a lot more money than my family did, and I felt like I was practically invisible around them.

FACILITATOR 2: How do you think this belief relates to smoking?

ALLISON: I started smoking at a young age, a really young age. I had my first drag when I was 8 years old—can you believe that? Eight! It was because I was with my older brother, and I wanted to fit in with his friends. Over the next few years, kids my age started smoking more and more—especially in my neighborhood, it seemed like *everyone* smoked. I guess I realized that smoking was one thing I could do in a group with other people. Before I knew it, I was included more often. You know, things like other kids asking me if I wanted to smoke a cigarette behind the dumpster with them after school.

FACILITATOR 1: Ah, so some of your basic beliefs are "I'm unlikable" and "I'm not good enough," and smoking counteracted those beliefs because others invited you to be part of their group?

ALLISON: Yeah, exactly.

ELLEN: Do you ever feel as depressed as I do, since that's the way you see yourself?

ALLISON: I've definitely struggled with depression in the past when things aren't going well. I know how it feels.

MICHAEL: Me too. I guess I also had some of that while growing up, with the way I didn't really fit in with the family.

FACILITATOR 2: And you were quite depressed when you first joined the group, when you thought your wife was going to leave you. Do you think these basic beliefs fueled your depression?

MICHAEL: I'm not sure I was really focused on people not caring or being unlikeable at that point. I just really felt like such a failure. I mean, I overcame growing up in a working class family where no one went to college, and even though education wasn't valued much in my home, I graduated from a good college, went to law school, and was hired by a great firm. When I first joined the group, it was about to all come crashing down. I thought I had lost everything, that I had failed in life.

FACILITATOR 1: You have just identified another basic belief that is often associated with depression—the belief that you are a failure. Has anyone else struggled with that belief?

DAVE: Don't ask me. I've never been depressed a day in my life. [Facilitator 1 chooses to move on from this comment because Dave is still relatively new to the group and often sends signals that he does not like to be pushed.]

BRIAN: That's exactly how I feel right now. Obviously, I've been attending sessions on a regular basis again, so you know what that means. A few weeks ago, I did it again. I fell into my old habits and blew the money I made doing a side job where I was paid under the table. I can't blame anyone but myself. I grew up with both of my parents, they were never divorced, I had a good childhood. I'm the one who pissed it away, and now my life is in the toilet because of it.

MICHAEL: Hang in there. I've been there before, too, and you've just got to keep focused on the prize—staying away from that stuff.

BRIAN: Thanks Michael. I appreciate what you're saying. But it seems pretty hopeless right now. I have nothing to show for my life.

ELLEN: But don't forget, Brian, that there *were* some aspects of your childhood that were difficult for you. Maybe your parents didn't drink or do drugs or abuse you, but I remember you saying that they were overly concerned with money and status. And because of that, they often gave you the sense that you weren't good enough.

BRIAN: I guess so. But, in the end, they were right. I wasn't good at school and ended up dropping out of a college no one had ever heard of, when my brother and sister graduated from good colleges and now have great careers. I have nothing.

FACILITATOR 1: (*gently*) Brian, would you say that you're feeling particularly depressed in the time since you've rejoined the group?

BRIAN: Yeah. I've started back up on meds.

FACILITATOR 1: It sounds like depression is a common experience for most of the group members. We'll be sure to work on strategies to manage depression in the future, OK?

BRIAN: OK.

FACILITATOR 1: (*turning to the entire group*) You all have done some great work here, work that I would, in fact, regard as essential. You've dug deep and identified powerful beliefs about yourselves and beliefs about the objects of your addiction that are fueling your addiction as well as depression. How might this information be useful to you?

MICHAEL: Well, in the past we've looked at our beliefs objectively, like looking at the evidence for and against them.

FACILITATOR 2: And what was the end result of doing that?

MICHAEL: I can't speak for everyone, but I know in my case, it helped me to see that I was focusing so much on my mistakes that I forgot about all of the other parts of me that make me a good person. That really helped me get through when I first joined the group.

ELLEN: Me too. If I can just remember not to blindly accept these beliefs when I'm all alone at home, it does me a lot of good.

FACILITATOR 1: Well, why don't we focus in on specific strategies for evaluating and modifying unhelpful beliefs. [Facilitators go on to implement some of the strategies described in Chapter 7.]

These vignettes illustrate the manner in which facilitators highlight the contributions of basic beliefs, addiction-related beliefs, early experiences, and early exposure to addictive behavior to addictive disorders. In addition, they highlight the intricate relation between addictions and psychiatric disorders, such as depression. Although these vignettes focused on these four main constructs from the distal background model of addiction, it should be recognized that facilitators can initiate similar lines of questioning about personality traits, other psychiatric symptoms or disorders, social support, and engagement in meaningful activities to advance group members' cognitive case conceptualizations. In most instances, facilitators not only create an environment for group members to consider the distal background factors that contribute to their addiction, but they also follow with one or more strategies described in Part II to begin to address them.

Proximal Situational Profile

The proximal situational profile compliments the distal background profile in that it captures the cognitive, behavioral, emotional, and physiological processes at work when group members are faced with an activating situation or trigger for their addictions. In contrast to the distal background profile, the proximal situational profile characterizes the thoughts that arise in *particular* situations and the manner in which they lead to *particular* behaviors. It is crucial for facilitators to generate proximal situational profiles that characterize the common anticipatory outcome expectancies, relief-oriented outcome expectancies, facilitating thoughts, and attentional biases that lead group members to engage in addictive behavior. In addition, facilitators consider the degree to which group members have beliefs of self-efficacy about their ability to manage triggers, urges, and cravings, as well as tangible coping strategies to do so. Figure 5.3 lists questions that are useful in constructing the proximal situational profile. The following vignette demonstrates the manner in which facilitators ask questions that elicit proximal situational profiles of some of the group members:

FACILITATOR 1: Who'd like to describe a situation in which they were faced with one or more triggers?

MICHAEL: I guess I can go. Last Friday at work, a bunch of the guys wanted to go out for drinks as soon as 5:00 rolled around. And guess where they wanted to go? (*Group members moan.*) You got it, a strip club.

FACILITATOR 1: So that was the trigger. What did you say to yourself?

- What kinds of "people, places, and things" trigger you to engage in addictive behavior?
- When faced with a trigger, what anticipatory outcome expectancies do you have about engaging in addictive behavior? Relief-oriented expectancies?
- When you think of [name of addiction], what runs through your mind?
- What do you expect will happen when you engage in addictive behavior?
- How do you give yourself permission to engage in addictive behavior?
- What are your urges and cravings like? What cognitive, emotional, and physiological sensations do you experience?
- How do you handle urges and cravings? How effective are those coping skills?
- How much do you believe you can refrain from engaging in addictive behavior when faced with a trigger?
- When you experience a trigger, urge, or craving, do you become consumed by it? How do you get your mind off of it?
- What are the consequences of your addictive behavior?
- What would life be like without [name of addiction]?

FIGURE 5.3. Sample questions to identify proximal situational factors.

MICHAEL: I actually had two different sets of thoughts. On the one hand, I was like, "I'm going to miss out if I don't go with the guys. I should go with them, or it will raise more questions than it's worth." You know, since I used to go with them all the time, no questions asked. But on the other hand, I said to myself, "I have come way too far to screw up now."

ELLEN: That's great that you could recognize the second thought, Michael. You've come a long way in this group.

BRIAN: Yeah, I should really try to learn from you.

FACILITATOR 2: This is the perfect example. The first thoughts you mentioned are examples of facilitating thoughts. Those are the ones that give us permission to engage in your addiction. If you *think* you are allowed to do something, or that you "should" do something, then you'll do it. But you also attempted to put the brakes on that thinking, by telling yourself how far you have come. Which set of thoughts eventually won out?

MICHAEL: The second set. I didn't do it. I was pretty torn. But I ended up concentrating on how far I've come, what I would lose if my wife found out, and I just drove home and focused on my kids the rest of the night until they went to bed.

FACILITATOR 1: What this demonstrates is that two different thoughts are associated with two very different courses of action. The thought "I've come way too far to screw up now" was associated with going home. *(turning to the group)* What behavior is associated with the thought, "I'm going to miss out?"

DAVE: Going to the strip club, I guess.

FACILITATOR 1: Right. So for you, 5:00 on Fridays is a trigger, especially when the other guys in the office are planning on going out. But you successfully combated your urge to join them with a new way of thinking.

This example highlights that the main types of cognitions associated with Michael's slips are facilitating thoughts (e.g., "I should go with them, or it will raise more questions than it's worth"). In contrast, other group members slip when they experience relief-oriented outcome expectancies. Consider the following vignette, which illustrates the interplay between facilitating thoughts and relief-oriented expectancies:

ALLISON: I guess I'm like Michael because I have facilitating thoughts. Like the other day, I was paying bills and balancing our checkbook. And once again, I realized that if we pay all of the bills in full, we'll only have a couple hundred left for the month—and we have to buy a month's worth of groceries on that! Whenever I get wound up over money, I'm like, "Oh God, I need a cigarette." And I always give in to it, saying it will be "just *one*."

FACILITATOR 1: I'm sorry to hear that you experience such distress when you are paying bills, Allison. And in this example you actually identified two types of thoughts that often facilitate addictive behavior. (*turning to the group*) Can anyone identify the two thoughts that Allison expressed?

ELLEN: Saying "I'll just have *one*" gives her permission?

FACILITATOR 1: You got it.

ELLEN: I figured that was it, since I often do the same thing with food. It will be OK if I only have *one* cookie, or one scoop of ice cream. Of course, it never ends up being just one.

BRIAN: Yeah, me too. It will be OK if I go to the casino and set my limit at $25. (*laughing sarcastically*) But I don't think I've *ever* gotten out with losing only $25.

ALLISON: I *am* able to keep it down to one, but what happens is that I'm more likely to give in and have "just one" the next time I'm stressed.

FACILITATOR 1: You have both identified two important consequences of facilitating thoughts. One is that having *one* of anything that is an addiction, whether it is a cigarette, a type of food, or a trip to the casino, is often a "foot in the door" that keeps the behavior going. Many people who struggle with addictions find that it's tough to stop after just having one. Although Allison is successful at only having one cigarette on a particular occasion, it sounds like it lowers the threshold for the future, such that it is even easier to decide to indulge in "just one." (*pausing*) What is the other type of thought that Allison expressed?

BRIAN: She said that she "needed a cigarette."

FACILITATOR 1: Right! What kind of a thought is that?

BRIAN: Um ... relief-oriented?

FACILITATOR 1: Right again! And what makes it a relief-oriented outcome expectancy?

BRIAN: I guess because she's stressed out because she's having trouble making ends meet, so smoking is a way to calm her down.

FACILITATOR 1: Excellent description. Allison, what do you think? Does this ring true for you?

ALLISON: It sure does. That's exactly what happens.

As was stated in Chapter 2, relief-oriented outcome expectancies are activated when a person is experiencing an aversive emotional state, and he or she seeks to reduce or eliminate it through the addictive behavior. Anticipatory outcome expectancies, in contrast, facilitate addictive behavior because the person hopes to experience something pleasurable, rather than avoid something aversive. Consider the following vignette, when it becomes clear that *both* anticipatory and relief-oriented outcome expectancies are operative in Dave's decision to go to the bar and drink alcohol with his friends:

FACILITATOR 2: Dave, how about you? What's one of your triggers for drinking?

DAVE: *(chuckling)* I don't need a trigger. I'm *always* up for drinking.

FACILITATOR 2: Fair enough. But are there certain situations where you are more likely to drink than others, or more likely to drink to the point of getting very drunk?

DAVE: I guess when I'm with my friends at the bar, especially if we start early, right after work.

FACILITATOR 2: OK, now we're getting somewhere. So your environment, being with friends at a bar right after work, is a potential trigger. When you're close to getting done with work, and you know your friends plan to meet up at the bar, what runs through your mind?

DAVE: I don't know, I just want to get there.

FACILITATOR 2: So you're looking forward to it. What if, for example, you were to see your friends after work but not drink?

DAVE: No way, it would suck if everyone was drinking except for me. Whenever we go out drinking, something really crazy seems to happen. We have a blast. *(pausing)* And enough things are going *wrong* in my life, that this is really something I can look forward to.

FACILITATOR 2: I'm sensing two kinds of outcome expectancies at work, Dave. On the one hand, you see drinking at the bar with friends to ensure a fun, exciting night. Is that right? *(Dave nods.)* We call that an anticipatory outcome expectancy, in that you're expecting good things to come from drinking. But I also sense that some relief-oriented outcome expectancies are operating as well, when you say that drinking with friends is something that you can look forward to amid the problems in your life. Might drinking with friends also be an *escape* for you?

DAVE: I guess so.

FACILITATOR 1: Has anyone else had a similar experience, such that you experienced both anticipatory and relief-oriented outcome expectancies? [Group proceeds to have a lively discussion about these expectancies.]

After obtaining information about triggers, anticipatory and relief-oriented expectancies, and facilitating thoughts, the facilitators link those situational and cognitive factors to urges and cravings, the decision to engage in the addictive behavior, and the implications for continued use or relapse. Facilitators might refer to a "vicious cycle" to illustrate the manner in which addiction-related cognitions often intensify urges and cravings and in which a slip creates additional triggers and stressors that increase one's vulnerability for relapse.

In addition to the cognitive behavioral sequence of events that occur when group members face a trigger, facilitators also keep alert for indicators of group members' self-efficacy and existing repertoire of coping strategies. Consider the following vignette, in which Brian continues to be down on himself about his ability to remain abstinent from gambling:

BRIAN: I think my situation is just hopeless. I have every single one of the thoughts that you all are talking about. I love the excitement of the casino. I probably gamble as a way to win money so that I can forget what a loser I am. And as soon as I come into any money, I give myself permission to go, thinking this will be the one time I'm gonna win big. (*shaking his head and putting his head in his hands*)

ELLEN: I know it *feels* hopeless, Brian. I feel like that, too, sometimes. But if you have even one victory, when you want to go to the casino and you stay away, you'll start to show yourself that you can do it. Look at how tough it was for Michael when he joined the group and how far he's come.

FACILITATOR 1: What you all are speaking to is something we call *self-efficacy*. I know we've talked about this in group before, probably before Dave and Allison joined. Does anyone remember what that term means?

MICHAEL: It's like confidence in yourself, right?

FACILITATOR 1: You got it. In the case of addiction, it's the confidence that you can cope successfully with a trigger and avoid a lapse.

BRIAN: I have zero confidence in myself right now.

FACILITATOR 1: Yes, I'm sensing that. What coping skills do you have in place to deal with triggers for gambling?

BRIAN: That's the problem. I don't think I have any, at least any that have actually worked.

FACILITATOR 1: *(turning to the group)* What coping skills have others used successfully in managing triggers, urges, or cravings?

[Group goes on to have a discussion about coping skills.]

DAVE: None of this really applies to me. I can stop drinking anytime I want. The problem is that I don't really *want* to stop drinking. Is there anything wrong with enjoying a beer now and then?

FACILITATOR 2: *(ignoring Dave's question for the moment, in order to continue to focus on coping rather than on the merits of abstinence versus controlled drinking)* So, for you, Dave, the issue is less about whether you believe you can stop drinking and more about your motivation to stop drinking.

DAVE: Yeah, I guess so.

BRIAN: I understand where you're coming from, Dave. I think that's part of the problem for me, I don't *really* want to stop, which, when you think about it, is kind of weird because gambling has caused me so many problems.

FACILITATOR 1: Fortunately, all of these issues can be addressed in the context of this group—coming to terms with where we are in our motivation to change, increasing our confidence in our ability to manage triggers, and developing coping skills. Of these three issues, which one does each of you think of as the most important to focus on today? [Facilitators go on to establish the focus of that day's group and the acquisition of cognitive and behavioral strategies.]

Assimilation of Information

Form 5.1 (at the end of the chapter) displays the CTAG Case Conceptualization Form. Facilitators can use this form to record the cognitive, behavioral, emotional, and social or environmental factors that contribute to the understanding of a group member's addictive behavior. There are three main parts of the form. The first two parts provide space for the facilitator to record information that is relevant to the components of the distal background and proximal situational profiles. The final part provides space for the facilitator to incorporate this information into a "working formulation," which is a narrative description that incorporates information from the distal background and proximal situational profiles to explain the pathway by which a group member's addictive behavior developed and is maintained. Six entries on the CTAG Case Conceptualization Form have asterisks—these pertain to the key cognitive content areas that perpetuate addictive behavior, including basic beliefs, addiction-related beliefs, anticipatory outcome expectancies, relief-oriented outcome expectancies, facilitating thoughts, and self-efficacy. Although any aspect of the cognitive case conceptualization can be and is targeted in the CTAG, it is these six areas that are often covered to the greatest extent in group sessions, as they are viewed as the core cognitive factors that facilitate addictive behavior. Figures 5.4–5.8 display the CTAG Case Conceptualization Forms for Ellen, Michael, Allison, Brian, and Dave, respectively.

FORMULATING THE COGNITIVE CASE CONCEPTUALIZATION OF THE GROUP

Unlike individual psychotherapy, group psychotherapy involves another layer of case conceptualization—conceptualization of the group as an entity. Figure 5.9 (on page 94) displays factors that facilitators consider when conceptualizing the group as a whole. Although there are individual differences in clinical presentations, there are also unifying themes relevant to most, if not all group members. This is the key to group conceptualization. These themes can be used to weave a coherent thread across sessions, to instill a sense of universality among group members, and to develop group cohesiveness.

CTAGs can be conceptualized according to many of the dimensions already discussed in this chapter, including commonalities in the development of addiction-related beliefs, activating situations or triggers, and slips and relapses. In the group highlighted in this chapter, we have seen that most group members had early experiences that set the stage for the development of basic beliefs, which in turn made them vulnerable to experiment with addictive behavior and receive a great deal of reinforcement for doing so. Moreover, all of the group members acknowledged certain situations or emotional states that make them vulnerable to slips and lapses. By understanding the entire group from the perspective of the comprehensive cognitive model of addiction, facilitators can highlight similarities in diverse clinical presentations, even when they are as different as the clinical presentations of Ellen and Dave. In fact, it is often helpful for the facilitator to explicitly point out these similarities to group members so that they will have insight into the many ways group discussion is relevant to their current situation and to the fundamental cognitive behavioral process of addiction that cuts across various substances and addictive behaviors. Consider the following vignette, which occurred after the discussion aimed at

(text resumes on page 95)

Name of Group Member: Ellen   **Date:** February 21, 2012

DISTAL BACKGROUND FACTORS

Family History: Mother was obese; two of eight siblings struggle with weight as adults

Relevant Personality Traits: Shyness

Current and Past Psychiatric Diagnoses: Current and recurrent major depressive disorder

Formative Experiences: Did not receive much attention from parents or peers

Early Exposure to and Experimentation with Addictions: Chronic use of sweets as comfort food

Social Support Network: Very limited; no close friends; little contact with children

Meaningful Activities: Very limited

*Unhelpful Basic Beliefs: I'm unlovable; I'm undesirable; no one cares about me

*Unhelpful Addiction-Related Beliefs: Food is my friend; I deserve enjoyment

PROXIMAL SITUATIONAL FACTORS

Triggers: Loneliness; boredom; holidays alone

*Anticipatory Outcome Expectancies: Sweets will give me pleasure

*Relief-Oriented Outcome Expectancies: I can't stand the way I feel

*Facilitating Thoughts: Just one is OK; nobody wants me, so it doesn't matter if I'm fat

Urges and Cravings (Type, Frequency, Intensity): Frequent sensitivity to hunger; mouth waters

(cont.)

FIGURE 5.4. Ellen's cognitive case conceptualization.

*Self-Efficacy: Little confidence that she can make positive changes in her life
Coping Strategies (Type, Helpfulness): Try to ignore cravings (unhelpful)
Attentional Biases: Commercials for food on television
Consequences of Addiction: Health problems; inability to work and move around
WORKING FORMULATION: Ellen's addiction stems from genetic factors and a predisposition toward depression, fueled by basic beliefs that she is unlovable and undesirable. Although she always struggled with these beliefs, they became particularly salient after her husband left her and her relationships with her children deteriorated. Currently, she views food as the only source of pleasure in her life, and she lacks the self-efficacy to make many positive changes in her life, including adhering to a diet and regular exercise program.

*Key cognitive areas that perpetuate addictive behaviors.

FIGURE 5.4. *(cont.)*

Name of Group Member: Michael   **Date:** February 21, 2012

DISTAL BACKGROUND FACTORS
Family History: Father had pornographic magazines around the house
Relevant Personality Traits: Overachiever
Current and Past Psychiatric Diagnoses: Past major depressive disorder
Formative Experiences: Perceived himself as an outsider, rejected by his family
Early Exposure to and Experimentation with Addictions: Began viewing pornography at age 15
Social Support Network: Relationship with wife strained; not close with family of origin

(cont.)

FIGURE 5.5. Michael's cognitive case conceptualization.

Meaningful Activities: *Career as an attorney; spending time with wife and children*
*Unhelpful Basic Beliefs: I'm inadequate; I'm not a man
*Unhelpful Addiction-Related Beliefs: I'm powerful; I'm a competent male

PROXIMAL SITUATIONAL FACTORS

Triggers: *Opportunities to have sex or view pornography (e.g., out-of-town business trip)*
*Anticipatory Outcome Expectancies: This will feel great
*Relief-Oriented Outcome Expectancies: This will relieve the tension that has been building up
*Facilitating Thoughts: I'm not having sex at home; I'm a man, and I can't help myself
Urges and Cravings (Type, Frequency, Intensity): Infrequent restlessness, agitation
*Self-Efficacy: After several months of treatment, confident that he can remain abstinent
Coping Strategies (Type, Helpfulness): Pro/con analysis, distraction (helpful)
Attentional Biases: Presence of an attractive female who shows interest in him
Consequences of Addiction: Wife does not trust him and has threatened divorce

WORKING FORMULATION: Michael grew up in a household in which he perceived that he was rejected by his father and brother because he did not share common interests. When he began to view pornographic magazines, he saw himself as powerful and a competent man. These views were reinforced by numerous casual relationships with desirable women. They became so central, and his behavior provided so much pleasure, that he risked his relationships with his wife and children to have extramarital affairs. He currently manages his sex addiction by focusing on long-term consequences of his behavior.

*Key cognitive areas that perpetuate addictive behaviors.

FIGURE 5.5. *(cont.)*

Name of Group Member: Allison   **Date:** February 21, 2012

DISTAL BACKGROUND FACTORS
Family History: Most family members smoked
Relevant Personality Traits: Complicity
Current and Past Psychiatric Diagnoses: Past major depressive disorder
Formative Experiences: Little supervision by parents; neglected by classmates
Early Exposure to and Experimentation with Addictions: Began smoking at age 8 to fit in
Social Support Network: Feels distant from coworkers and family members who smoke
Meaningful Activities: Spending time with children; needlepoint
*Unhelpful Basic Beliefs: I'm not good enough; I'm unlikable
*Unhelpful Addiction-Related Beliefs: Smoking is cool; I fit in with the crowd
PROXIMAL SITUATIONAL FACTORS
Triggers: Husband and mother-in-law smoke in house; situational stressors (e.g., bills)
*Anticipatory Outcome Expectancies: None
*Relief-Oriented Outcome Expectancies: A cigarette will help me get through this
*Facilitating Thoughts: Just one is OK; If I can't beat them, I might as well join them
Urges and Cravings (Type, Frequency, Intensity): Frequent irritability, restlessness

(cont.)

FIGURE 5.6. Allison's cognitive case conceptualization.

*Self-Efficacy: Believes she is successful at some tasks, but quitting smoking is overwhelming

Coping Strategies (Type, Helpfulness): Nicotine gum, patch (variable helpfulness)

Attentional Biases: Other people smoking around her

Consequences of Addiction: Increased risk for lung cancer; coughing; trouble breathing

WORKING FORMULATION: Allison's addiction stems from early exposure to cigarettes by family and peers. As a neglected child, she believed that she was unlikeable, and smoking helped her to fit in with the crowd. Although those anticipatory outcome expectancies are no longer at work, she experiences powerful relief-oriented expectancies, urges, and cravings when she is in the presence of others who smoke, which occurs frequently. Allison generally regards herself as an effective person but is having difficulty applying this self-efficacy to her nicotine addiction.

*Key cognitive areas that perpetuate addictive behaviors.

FIGURE 5.6. *(cont.)*

Name of Group Member: Brian   **Date:** February 21, 2012

DISTAL BACKGROUND FACTORS

Family History: Family members did not gamble; alcoholism on father's side of the family

Relevant Personality Traits: Lack of reward sensitivity

Current and Past Psychiatric Diagnoses: Current major depressive disorder

Formative Experiences: Family placed excessive importance on money and status

Early Exposure to and Experimentation with Addictions: Began to gamble at age 21

Social Support Network: Wife considering divorce; parents disappointed in him

(cont.)

FIGURE 5.7. Brian's cognitive case conceptualization.

Meaningful Activities: Limited—working several side jobs to make money

*Unhelpful Basic Beliefs: I am a failure; I am incompetent

*Unhelpful Addiction-Related Beliefs: Winning makes me successful.

PROXIMAL SITUATIONAL FACTORS
Triggers: Coming into money unexpectedly

*Anticipatory Outcome Expectancies: Winning big gives me a high

*Relief-Oriented Outcome Expectancies: This will make me forget about what a loser I am

*Facilitating Thoughts: It will all be OK if I just win

Urges and Cravings (Type, Frequency, Intensity): Preoccupation with gambling and winning big

*Self-Efficacy: Little confidence that he can make positive changes in his life

Coping Strategies (Type, Helpfulness): None

Attentional Biases: Money in his wallet

Consequences of Addiction: Financial instability; wife may divorce him

WORKING FORMULATION: Brian was raised in a household in which money and status were viewed as essential features of being successful. Because Brian struggled academically, he developed the basic belief that he is a failure and is incompetent. Soon after he turned 21, he began gambling. In addition to giving him a "high," it taught him that he can attain large sums of money quickly. However, he has trouble knowing when to stop, and his gambling almost always causes adverse consequences. He does not believe that he can make money (and, thereby, achieve status) in any other way.

*Key cognitive areas that perpetuate addictive behaviors.

FIGURE 5.7. *(cont.)*

Name of Group Member: Dave   **Date:** February 21, 2012

DISTAL BACKGROUND FACTORS
Family History: Father and many extended family members had alcohol and drug problems
Relevant Personality Traits: Lack of empathy; self-centeredness; impulsivity
Current and Past Psychiatric Diagnoses: Possible antisocial personality disorder
Formative Experiences: Circle of friends got in trouble at school and with the law
Early Exposure to and Experimentation with Addictions: Used alcohol and drugs at a young age
Social Support Network: Volatile relationship with girlfriend; all friends are users
Meaningful Activities: Very limited
*Unhelpful Basic Beliefs: People should look out for themselves; no one cares
*Unhelpful Addiction-Related Beliefs: This is how I have fun; this makes problems go away
PROXIMAL SITUATIONAL FACTORS
Triggers: Being around friends who use; argument with girlfriend
*Anticipatory Outcome Expectancies: I'm gonna get wasted and have a great night
*Relief-Oriented Outcome Expectancies: This will help me to forget my problems
*Facilitating Thoughts: All of my friends do it, so why shouldn't I?
Urges and Cravings (Type, Frequency, Intensity): Daily preoccupation with alcohol and drugs

(cont.)

FIGURE 5.8. Dave's cognitive case conceptualization.

*Self-Efficacy: Believes he can stop using anytime he wants to do so
Coping Strategies (Type, Helpfulness): None
Attentional Biases: End of the work day
Consequences of Addiction: Difficulty holding down job; conflict with girlfriend
WORKING FORMULATION: Dave's addiction stems from a genetic predisposition and early exposure to multiple people in his life who abused alcohol and drugs. He experimented with alcohol and drugs at an early age, and his deviant lifestyle prevented him from obtaining positive reinforcement through other means. Dave has the basic belief that people should look out for themselves, so he does not consider the consequences of his addiction on others. He is currently in the precontemplation stage of change and has yet to develop effective coping skills to manage his addictive behaviors.

*Key cognitive areas that perpetuate addictive behaviors.

FIGURE 5.8. Dave's cognitive case conceptualization.

COMMON COGNITIVE BEHAVIORAL PROCESSES
• Basic beliefs
• Addiction-related beliefs
• Outcome expectancies
• Facilitating thoughts
• Self-efficacy and coping
• Triggers
• Responses to slips and lapses
READINESS FOR CHANGE
• Length of time members have been in the group
• Degree of motivation to make changes in life
• Opportunity for group members to model coping to one another
TRUST AND COHESIVENESS

FIGURE 5.9. Information included in the group cognitive case conceptualization.

developing group members' distal background and the proximal situational profiles:

FACILITATOR 1: You all have worked hard today. It's not easy to reach back and conjure up all of those basic beliefs, many of which are quite painful. I'd like to summarize what we've learned about the cognitive model to understanding addictions, which I think will help you to solidify and apply what we've done so far in group and what we'll continue to do in the future. So, who'd like to tell me what they learned about addictions today?

ALLISON: I can say that I've learned a lot, since I haven't been in group that long and hadn't had the chance to think about my situation in these terms.

FACILITATOR 1: Glad to hear that this has been helpful, Allison. How would you explain the cognitive model of addiction?

ALLISON: I'd say that a lot of things go into addictions, not just being weak or passive, like I had thought. In my case, being ignored by the other kids made me feel badly about myself. So when I had the chance to start smoking, I didn't think twice because it made me feel like I was part of a group. Now, though, smoking has become a habit for me, and I use it more when I need relief from all of the stress.

FACILITATOR 1: Excellent description, Allison. You've identified several of the major components—early experiences, basic beliefs, the manner in which they contributed to the development of addiction-related beliefs, and the types of thoughts and expectancies that operate now when you experience urges and cravings. What I'd like to emphasize is the commonality of your experiences, despite the fact that you all have very different backgrounds and struggle with very different addictions. For example, the relief-oriented expectancy of wanting to escape or reduce stress is something I've heard from most, if not all of you. Ellen has urges to eat when she is confronted with her problems, Allison has urges to smoke when she is confronted with her problems, Brian has urges to gamble when he is confronted with his problems, and Dave has urges to drink when he is confronted with his problems. What this suggests to me is that even when one of you brings up a specific problem in your life, the *process* of how the problem arises, how it affects urges, cravings, slips, and lapses, and how it affects your mood and well-being are similar. I will be sure to point out the underlying process in future groups so that you can think about how one member's problem might apply to your own, even if on the surface the problem seems very different.

CTAGs also can be conceptualized according to their readiness for change. Although each group member will, undoubtedly, be in a unique stage of change, the group itself also can vary according to its openness to various types of interventions. For example, some newer members might not yet have acquired many cognitive and behavioral coping strategies, but they are motivated to make positive changes in their lives and have made a commitment to abstinence. Some more seasoned group members, in contrast, might have had more exposure to cognitive and behavioral coping strategies, but, like Brian, they are less committed to change and often experience slips and lapses. Still other group members are veterans and are in the maintenance stage of change, in which they might not be practicing the cognitive and behavioral coping strategies as actively because they have adopted a new lifestyle, free of their addiction. Facilitators must balance group members' stage of change, experience with cognitive and behavioral coping strategies, and history of success and failure in choosing interventions and in highlighting problems experienced by certain group members that would have the most relevance for others.

We can provide numerous examples of the manner in which the composition of the group determines the specific interventions that facilitators select. Consider, for example, a group composed of a few seasoned veterans who have made positive changes in their lives for some time and several newer members. If those newer members are a bit skeptical of the group and are in the precontemplation or contemplation stages of change, then the group might benefit from the seasoned veterans sharing their successes. Not only will these success stories demonstrate to the newer members that change is possible (i.e., instillation of hope), but they will also allow the seasoned veterans an opportunity to enhance their self-worth by reflecting on their success and serving as positive role models for newer members (i.e., imparting of information, increasing self-efficacy). In contrast, suppose the newer members are in the action stage of change and are committed to "making the most" out of the CTAG. These newer members are ripe for instruction on *how* to make positive changes in their lives; thus, facilitators might encourage the seasoned veterans to describe the cognitive and behavioral coping strategies that were most useful for them in more detail, and to explain why they were useful. Then, facilitators might encourage group members to actively practice one or more of these skills in session.

Most often, groups consist of members with a wide variety of experience with the group, stages of change, and experience with success and failure. Some of those individuals will be positive, motivating influences on the group, whereas, at times, there will be other individuals whose negative attitude toward treatment interferes with the group's ability to make use of the material that is being discussed. Facilitators can work strategically to maximize the influence of the group members with positive attitudes in order to create a group atmosphere oriented toward support and change.

Take Dave, as an example. In some of the vignettes provided earlier in this chapter, Dave presented as irritable at times and questioned the relevance of some of the material that the facilitators were presenting. The facilitators used this information to hypothesize that Dave is in the precontemplation stage of change and that there is a potential for Dave to disrupt the group with his negative attitude. On the basis of these hypotheses, the facilitators (1) chose not to highlight Dave's problems in public if he did not volunteer them; (2) chose not to push Dave if he did not communicate a readiness to apply the cognitive model to his own problems; (3) used a welcoming, nondefensive tone when Dave questioned the material; and (4) highlighted the similarities between Dave's problems and other group members'. As a result, despite Dave's resistance, the group was open to frank discussion and the acquisition of new cognitive and behavioral coping strategies, and Dave was implicitly given permission to take home the material that he thought was relevant to him. As is seen in subsequent chapters, Dave continued to attend the group, and although he also continued to have an "edge" to him, he assumed a greater readiness to change as treatment progressed.

Thus, the group's openness to strategic intervention is dependent not only on the group members' individual differences, but also on the manner in which the facilitator handles those differences. In our experience, even groups composed mainly of new members who have not yet reached the action stage of change are open to many topics of discussion if the positive attitudes and successes of group members are acknowledged, differences of opinion are respected, and the similarities are identified and conceptualized by the facilitators.

Finally, groups can be conceptualized according to the degree of trust and cohesiveness that they exhibit. Many group members report that the group's greatest value is the support given and received by fellow members. Although facilitators should be skillful in providing feedback to group members, often, feedback is most meaningful when it comes from another group member. However, facilitators must approach feedback among group members with caution, as negative feedback that is presented in an abrupt manner has the potential to shame the group member in public and lead to that individual slipping or never returning to group. Facilitators can use principles of modeling to demonstrate effective strategies for providing feedback, first by providing feedback themselves, and then by providing positive reinforcement to group members who provide appropriate feedback. In the event that a fellow group member provides excessively negative or inappropriate feedback, the facilitator can use many of the strategies described in Chapter 8 (e.g., effective communication) to address the issue and turn it into a positive learning experience for all.

SUMMARY

The cognitive case conceptualization plays a pivotal role in the CTAG, as (1) it helps the facilitator to understand group members' clinical presentations in light of the comprehensive cognitive model of addiction, (2) it allows the facilitator to generate hypotheses about the factors that maintain group members' emotional and behavioral disturbances, and (3) it guides the selection of specific interventions. In CTAGs, the facilitator constructs two layers of cognitive case conceptualizations—conceptualizations of individual group members' clinical presentations, and a conceptualization of the group as a whole. Information that is used to formulate individual case conceptualizations includes distal background factors that make group members vulnerable to engage in addictive behavior and proximal situational variables that explain the cognitive and behavioral factors at work when group members are confronted with a trigger. Often, facilitators obtain this information when group members describe their problems, when they introduce themselves to the group, or when the facilitator educates group members about the cognitive model. Facilitators attempt to ask questions that will aid in the construction of the cognitive case conceptualization of many members simultaneously. However, because facilitators might not be able to obtain in-depth information from any one group member at any one time, many aspects of the conceptualization are formed as hypotheses to be modified as more information is gathered. The cognitive case conceptualization of the group as a whole incorporates similarities in group members' distal background and proximal situational profiles, group members' readiness for change, and the degree of trust and cohesiveness that characterizes the group.

Cognitive case conceptualizations help facilitators to select interventions that will be most useful in modifying unhelpful beliefs, managing urges and cravings, and assisting group members in developing cognitive and behavioral coping skills. In many instances, a general intervention will be selected that targets one aspect of the cognitive model, and each member will implement a specific strategy on the basis of his or her unique beliefs and/or life circumstances. These interventions and specific strategies are described in Part II.

FORM 5.1. CTAG Case Conceptualization Form

Name of Group Member: _____ **Date:** _____

DISTAL BACKGROUND FACTORS
Family History:
Relevant Personality Traits:
Current and Past Psychiatric Diagnoses:
Formative Experiences:
Early Exposure to and Experimentation with Addictions:
Social Support Network:
Meaningful Activities:
*Unhelpful Basic Beliefs:
*Unhelpful Addiction-Related Beliefs:

(cont.)

PROXIMAL SITUATIONAL FACTORS
Triggers:
*Anticipatory Outcome Expectancies:
*Relief-Oriented Outcome Expectancies:
*Facilitating Thoughts:
Urges and Cravings (Type, Frequency, Intensity):
*Self-Efficacy:
Coping Strategies (Type, Helpfulness):
Attentional Biases:
Consequences of Addiction:
WORKING FORMULATION:

*Key cognitive areas that perpetuate addictive behaviors.

PART II COGNITIVE THERAPY ADDICTIONS GROUP SESSION COMPONENTS

INTRODUCTION TO PART II

Conducting group psychotherapy is stimulating, rewarding, and challenging for facilitators as they promote group cohesiveness and manage the needs and personalities of individual group members while simultaneously remaining mindful of the needs of the group as a whole. In group cognitive therapy, an additional dimension to consider is the balance between attending to group cohesiveness and promoting cognitive and behavioral change. Cognitive and behavioral change can be fostered through a number of different pathways, such as by providing psychoeducation, allowing group members to practice strategies in session, and encouraging group members to learn from one another.

Part II contains four chapters that correspond to different segments of the CTAG. In Chapter 6, readers learn the procedure for facilitating the introductions that take place at the beginning of a group session. Readers are provided with examples of ways to identify themes that cut across the concerns that group members introduce, as well as ways to integrate new members into the group. In Chapter 7, readers learn strategies for modifying situational thoughts and underlying beliefs. Readers are exposed to ways to apply these strategies specific to addiction-related thoughts and beliefs, as well as thoughts and beliefs associated with emotional distress. In Chapter 8, readers learn a large array of coping skills that they can share with group members as they are indicated and have group members practice in session. In Chapter 9, readers gain a sense of the manner in which homework logically follows from the work done in session and ways to maximize homework compliance. In addition, this chapter provides readers with strategies for attaining closure at the end of a session and different scenarios that may arise during the closure process. After reading Part II, readers come away with knowledge of how to conduct CTAGs and specific strategies they can use that have the potential to decrease the likelihood that group members will relapse and increase the likelihood that they can manage their emotional distress and interpersonal problems.

CHAPTER 6 | Introductions

Introductions are an important part of CTAGs because they set the tone for the remainder of the session. When facilitators introduce themselves, their tone of voice, posture, and eye contact communicate that they are respectful of the difficulties group members have experienced, and at the same time, that they are competent in treating a range of addictions. Group members' introductions model to other members that each person who is in the group continues to experience the consequences of his or her addictive behavior, that some degree of active participation is expected, and that members will be attentive and respectful toward others. Facilitators listen carefully to themes that emerge from group members' introductions and use those opportunities to educate the group about the cognitive model of addiction, and later, guide the acquisition of cognitive and behavioral strategies to manage addiction and lead a discussion of other issues that are relevant to associated psychiatric symptoms and well-being.

FACILITATOR INTRODUCTIONS

CTAG facilitators introduce themselves by stating their name and why they facilitate the group. They also may include brief but relevant professional information, such as the length of time they have been employed in that particular setting or the length of time they have been working with individuals who struggle with addictions. Because facilitators' introductions serve as models for the remaining introductions, they should be carefully considered. If facilitators' introductions are shallow or superficial, group members will probably respond with similarly superficial introductions. In contrast, if facilitators are warm, honest, spontaneous, and engaging during their introductions, then group members are likely to respond in kind.

As was stated earlier in this volume, on occasion, group members will ask facilitators about their own recovery status, as many individuals with addictions have the false belief that only someone who struggled with addictions him- or herself is able to provide effective treatment. We recommend that facilitators carefully weigh the advantages and disadvantages of self-disclosure and do so only in instances in which such disclosure would facilitate authenticity and group cohesiveness. Facilitators should not actively initiate discussions about their own addictive behavior in order to maintain appropriate boundaries. Thus, when self-disclosure regarding facilitators' histories with addictive behaviors occurs, it should be only in response to group members' inquiries, and excessive detail should be avoided.

After facilitators introduce themselves, they describe the structure, content, and rules of the group. The *structure* of the group includes those elements described in Chapter 4, including introductions, cognitive and behavioral strategies, development of a homework assignment, and closure. The *content* of the group is determined by the concerns introduced by group members during the introductions, such as dealing with urges and cravings, managing symptoms of depression and anxiety, or developing skills to address problems in their close relationships. The cognitive model of addictions is reviewed in every session, and other content areas introduced by group members are understood from a cognitive behavioral perspective. The *rules* of the group are guidelines for participation. As was stated in Chapter 4, one basic rule is confidentiality—group members are asked to refrain from discussing the specific details of group outside of the session and to not reveal the identities of other individuals in the group. Another basic rule is that group members should not attend a session under the influence of alcohol or drugs. In addition, group members are asked to (1) be respectful and considerate of one another; (2) be as honest, open, and specific about their own situation as much as possible, rather than philosophizing or generalizing; and (3) minimize disruptions (e.g., by turning off cell phones). The following example illustrates a facilitator introduction:

> "Hello, my name is Bruce, and I have facilitated this CTAG for over 15 years. I am a licensed clinical psychologist who has been working in the field of addictions ever since I graduated from graduate school. I facilitate this group because it is very gratifying for me, as I have seen many group members over the years who have made tremendous changes in their lives. [*Structure:*] Each session of this group follows the same structure. After giving my introduction, I will ask each of you to take up to 5 minutes and introduce yourself. Tell us your name,

your past and present addictions, the status of your addictions, your goals, and any other concerns or issues you might have. [*Content:*] The topics discussed in group will depend partly on the concerns you raise in your introductions. Regardless of the specific topic under consideration, all group sessions will include a discussion of cognitive and behavioral strategies that can be applied to the issues with which you are struggling. [*Rules:*] I'd like to mention a few simple ground rules for the group. First, keep all information about this group confidential. This means that I'd like you to refrain from sharing anything you hear about others in this group with outsiders, including the names of other group members. Second, don't show up for group under the influence of alcohol or drugs, as that has the potential to be very disruptive to other group members who are working hard to manage their own addiction. Third, treat others considerately and respectfully, as you would like to be treated. Fourth, talk honestly and personally about yourself rather than philosophizing, generalizing, or talking about others. For example, instead of using phrases like 'I know that smoking has negative effects on people's health,' describe how smoking has had a negative effect on *your* health. And finally, please minimize any disruptions during the session. Turning off your cell phone would be one way to do this. Does anyone have any questions or anything to add?"

If there are a number of new members in the group, it is often helpful to provide a context for the use of a group cognitive approach. For example, facilitators might describe evidence suggesting that cognitive and behavioral strategies are useful in treating addictive behaviors as well as in treating associated symptoms of depression, anxiety, and relationship distress (see Chapter 1). Facilitators could also describe the manner in which participation in CTAGs is complementary to participation in 12-step programs and highlight the group processes that are at work in both settings. If facilitators choose to mention this in their introductions, they should take care to indicate that participation in a 12-step program is in no way a prerequisite for participation in the CTAG and that the opinions of group members who choose not to participate in 12-step programs are respected. In addition, facilitators can provide a more detailed and personalized account of the manner in which he or she has witnessed the group's positive influence on members. Such strategies serve to increase group members' confidence in this approach and instill hope that they will have success.

In sum, facilitator introductions serve a number of purposes. At the most fundamental level, they set group members' expectations for the structure, content, and rules of the group. However, they also set the tone for the nature of the interactions among group members, in that their verbal and nonverbal behaviors promote an environment of warmth, empathy, and support, as well as one that provides tangible education about the coping strategies that are expected to make a difference in group members' lives. It is hoped that the content and tone of facilitators' introductions create a welcoming environment for group members, begin to relieve anxiety about sharing in a group format, and instill hope that group members' addictions and other problems can be addressed successfully.

GROUP MEMBER INTRODUCTIONS

After facilitators introduce themselves, group members introduce themselves by stating their name, past and present addictions, status of each of their addictions, goals, and other issues. Facilitators often set a precise amount of time that each person can take for his or her introduction, such as 2 minutes per introduction in very large groups (i.e., 10 to 12 people), or more typically (as stated in the sample facilitator introduction), 5 minutes per introduction. It is important for facilitators to balance allowing enough time for the group member to express his or her concerns with ensuring that introductions are not so lengthy that other group members become bored or disengaged. Regardless of the specific amount of time decided upon by facilitators, it is important that they follow through with implementing that convention so that each group member is treated equally, and also so that the use of unstructured time is not inadvertently reinforced in instances in which group members run far over time in their introduction.

Introductions provide the first opportunity for group members to learn vicariously from one another. In every session, they hear about the successful and unsuccessful ways in which members have attempted to cope with their addictive behaviors. During introductions, group cohesiveness begins to develop as members share their problems, struggles, setbacks, and plans for improving their lives. As group members introduce themselves, one of the facilitators completes the CTAG Attendance and Summary Form, presented in Form 6.1 (at the end of the chapter). This form allows the facilitator to document the symptoms and problems described by group members and organize this information in a meaningful way. Moreover, because the group will choose a topic to discuss later in the session, the CTAG Attendance and Summary Form serves as a quick guide for helping facilitators to identify the topic of relevance to the most group members.

The following vignette provides a typical example of members' introductions. The facilitators have already introduced themselves and have asked group members to state their name, addictions, status, goals, and other issues. As group members talk, their responses are noted on Facilitator 2's CTAG Attendance and Summary Form (see Figure 6.1):

FACILITATOR 1: Who wants to start with their introduction?

MICHAEL: I guess I'll go first. My name is Michael, and I have a sex addiction. I haven't had any slips in 6 months. Things seem to be going better now, at least to some degree, with my wife and kids.

FACILITATOR 1: So Michael, you have a sex addiction, but you've been abstinent for awhile now. Congratulations on that. (*Group members nod and give the "thumbs-up" sign in approval.*) What's your goal for the future?

MICHAEL: Staying away from anything related to sex—other women, strip clubs, porn movies, *Playboys*. It's poison and almost cost me my family.

FACILITATOR 2: Any other issues of concern?

MICHAEL: Not really, I just want to learn as much as I can so that I can do whatever it takes to keep my family together.

FACILITATOR 1: OK, who wants to go next?

(*Silence for about 5 seconds*)

ALLISON: I guess I can go. Since I've only been to one group so far, I wasn't sure if I should wait for other people to go before me.

FACILITATOR 2: We appreciate your sensitivity to the group process, Allison. But you can be assured that all members are considered equal, no matter how long they have been attending group.

ALLISON: OK, well that's a relief. Hi, my name is Allison, and this is my second week with this group so that I can finally stop smoking once and for all.

FACILITATOR 1: And your status?

ALLISON: I cut down big time right after I had a doctor's appointment, and she told me that I already have some bad effects of smoking on my lungs and that my health will continue to go downhill if I don't quit. Some days I don't even smoke one cigarette. But, boy, it has been tough. My husband and his mother both keep smoking in the house, so I am always around it. So that gives me cravings. And then I also worry about the effects of their secondhand smoke, since my lungs are already messed up.

FACILITATOR 1: That sounds like a tough situation. And you said you want to quit smoking once and for all ... does that mean forever?

ALLISON: Forever!

FACILITATOR 2: Any other issues that have been bothering you?

ALLISON: Well, I also want to learn stuff to make my family relationships better. I don't think my husband and mother-in-law

Group Member's Name	Addictions (Past and Present)	Status of Addictive Behaviors	Goals (e.g., Abstinence, Reduction)	Other Issues
Member 1 Dave	Alcohol	Daily use	Reduction, but still "have fun"	Conflict with girlfriend
	Marijuana	Regular use	Reduction, but still "have fun"	
	Crack cocaine	Occasional use	Abstinence (unconvincing)	
Member 2 Michael	Sex, pornography	6 months of abstinence	Continued abstinence	Cravings Re-establishing healthy relationships with family
Member 3 Ellen	Overeating	Regular overeating	Lose 100 lbs. regular exercise routine abstinence from overeating	Depression Loneliness
Member 4 Allison	Cigarettes	2 weeks of near abstinence	Full abstinence	Cravings Tension with family members Health issues
Member 5 Brian	Gambling	Recent lapse	Abstinence (unconvincing)	Conflict with wife Financial problems Potential housing problems

FIGURE 6.1. Sample of a completed CTAG Attendance and Summary Form.

understand what I am going through, and the fact that they keep smoking around me certainly doesn't help. They won't listen to me whenever I ask them to smoke outside. Now we're all in a big fight, and I dread coming home after work.

FACILITATOR 1: Thanks for sharing, Allison. It's sounding as if a theme might be emerging today—problems with relationships. That's a common problem among people with addictions—conflict with others who either have been hurt by the addiction or who are unsupportive as you try to kick the addiction. What do you think? (*Most group members nod.*) Before we get to that, though, let's see what's going on with Ellen.

ELLEN: I'm Ellen, and I think I have the opposite problem. I don't have any relationship conflicts right now, but it's because I don't really talk regularly to anyone in my family. I feel like I'm all by myself and just a big nothing. (*becomes tearful*)

FACILITATOR 1: (*gently*) It sounds like relationship problems also apply to you, just in a different way than what we heard from Michael and Allison. Ellen, can you share your addiction, status, and goals?

ELLEN: (*sniffing*) My addiction is overeating. Even though I've been coming to group for 6 months now, I really haven't done anything about it. I really want to, and my doctor tells me that I better change my eating habits, or I will have major health problems. But it's just so hard right now. I'm stuck in that tiny apartment all alone, and I feel so lonely and bored that eating is really the only thing I have to look forward to.

FACILITATOR 1: So it sounds like you're still trying to get your addiction under control. What is your ultimate goal?

ELLEN: Well, the doctor says I need to lose 100 pounds. And start exercising. I have no idea how to do that though; I can barely walk up one flight of stairs without losing my breath.

FACILITATOR 2: You also mentioned loneliness and lack of communication with your family—is it safe to say those are other issues? Are there any other issues with which you are struggling?

ELLEN: No, I guess all of this is just making me feel really depressed.

FACILITATOR 2: OK, depression.... Ellen, thanks for sharing all of that with us; I realize you are going through a difficult time now. Who would like to go next in introductions?

DAVE: (*large sigh*) My name is Dave. Not David—I hate it when people call me that. I drink and smoke weed a lot. I got a DUI awhile ago and ended up in jail.

FACILITATOR 1: OK, your addictions are marijuana and alcohol, anything else?

DAVE: (*slightly irritated*) Well, I also snort coke every once in a while, but I don't know if it would be considered an addiction because it isn't very often, and I don't think it causes any more problems than the other stuff.

FACILITATOR 1: You mentioned that your addictions landed you in jail with a DUI. Are there any other negative consequences to your addictions?

DAVE: Well, I guess my girlfriend gets real mad that I use, which leads to a lot of fights. But I also have a lot of fun with my friends when I'm using, and it gets me away from the constant nagging at home.

FACILITATOR 1: And the current status of your addiction?

DAVE: I had a real good time with my buddies a couple of nights ago. But I think I'm cutting down some. Like last night, after work I just chilled with a couple of beers and went to bed.

FACILITATOR 2: What are your goals for your addictions?

DAVE: I guess I should cut down—I could get in a lot of trouble if I get another DUI. But I still want to let loose and have fun every once in a while, I guess drink and light up a joint from time to time.

FACILITATOR 2: What is your goal for cocaine?

DAVE: Well, like I said, I don't really see that as a problem. But I was thinking of stopping that anyway because it's so damn expensive. My girlfriend keeps bitching at me that we need to save money for a new car now that I totaled our old one.

FACILITATOR 2: So you are considering abstinence for your cocaine use?

DAVE: Yeah, sure, I guess so.

FACILITATOR 1: Do you have any other issues that are concerning you?

DAVE: I don't know, nothing really. I guess I'd just like my girlfriend to get off my back so I can relax when I get home from work, you know?

FACILITATOR 1: It sounds like you also are having some relationship difficulties and could benefit from developing some skills to communicate with your girlfriend.

DAVE: I guess, it would be nice to know how to tell her to leave me alone and have it actually stick!

FACILITATOR 1: Communication, in one form or another, is something that most, if not all of us, can stand to work on. Before we move on, Brian, can we check in with you?

BRIAN: I'm Brian, I have a gambling addiction. And I have big problems with my wife because of it.

FACILITATOR 1: Another instance of relationship problems related to an addiction. What is the status of and goals for your addiction?

BRIAN: I just keep going in this endless cycle. I quit for a while, sometimes several months on end. But then I get some extra money, and it's like all of those months don't mean anything.

FACILITATOR 2: (*gently*) So, for how long have you been able to stay away from gambling?

BRIAN: (*shaking head and looking glum*) Not long at all. I just lost thousands of dollars a few weeks ago, which I got from working my ass off on some extra contracting work and which I had promised to my wife to put a big down payment on a new car.

FACILITATOR 2: Sounds like you are going through a tough time.

BRIAN: Yeah, you don't know the half of it.

FACILITATOR 2: What is your goal for your addiction?

BRIAN: (*dejected*) I'd like to stay away from gambling, but I don't know how.

FACILITATOR 1: Well, that's what this group is all about. Any other issues?

BRIAN: (*sarcastically*) You mean besides the fact that my wife is about to leave me, we're in serious debt, and we're about to lose our home?

FACILITATOR 1: Sounds like you have a lot on your plate, and I'm hopeful that you'll be able to take away something tangible to address one of these problems by the end of today's session.

As illustrated in this vignette, the facilitator summarizes common themes, problems, and issues that arise during group member introductions. Facilitators balance giving fairly equal time for each group member to provide a brief status update, providing hope and encouragement, and identifying possible directions for the remainder of the group session.

Integrating New Members into the CTAG

As has been stated previously in this volume, the CTAG is an open group, meaning that people can attend as many or as few sessions as they see fit. Because of this characteristic, members enter and exit on a regular basis, and each session has the potential to be an "initial session" for one or more members. Thus, facilitators must have a plan for acclimating new members into the group, and conversely, for working with existing group members to welcome new people and secure their own place in the group. The first session of the CTAG may be the most important session that a group member attends. Not only are new members socialized into the structure and process of the CTAG during the first session, but they also develop initial impressions and attitudes about the group and its potential benefits.

There are advantages and disadvantages associated with the open nature of the group. Advantages include the regular infusion of new group members, which is likely to stimulate new perspectives and coping strategies. New members also enable seasoned group members to review the cognitive model of addiction and cognitive and behavioral concepts from a fresh perspective. Additionally, existing group members have the opportunity to be altruistic, offer support and encouragement to the newcomers, and act as "cheerleaders." The presence of new members allows existing group members to clearly see the progress they have made and to experience a renewed sense of accomplishment. Furthermore, addiction treatments often suffer from high drop-out rates (cf. Dutra et al., 2008), sometimes as high as 60–70% (Malat et al., 2008; Tzilos, Rhodes, Ledgerwood, & Greenwald, 2009). An open format allows groups to keep running strong. In contrast, one main disadvantage of the open-ended nature of the group is that some new members (particularly those who are especially quiet, labile, or oppositional) may inhibit disclosure by existing group members or disrupt cohesiveness.

In Chapter 4, we mention that we strongly encourage that facilitators have an individual meeting with potential new members before they attend their group session. Although the rules and basis for the group are reviewed in each session, it is helpful for potential new members to have this information in advance so that they can take some time to digest it and evaluate whether the group is right for them. In addition, an individual meeting with potential group members helps the facilitator to identify any factors that would preclude participation in group sessions, such as active psychotic symptoms or acute suicidal or homicidal ideation. In these cases, the facilitator is able to devote his or her full attention to the potential new group member in the individual meeting and make appropriate referrals. Finally, the individual meeting is useful for the facilitator to gather information that will help him or her to formulate an initial cognitive case conceptualization of the potential group member's clinical presentation. At the end of the individual meeting, it is important for the facilitator to solicit feedback from the potential new group members so that they can evaluate whether the group is a good fit for them, and so that they have a sense that they are already active participants and that their feedback is valued. Thus, the individual meeting begins to model the group process that a new member will observe during his or her first session.

Figure 6.2 lists strategies for integrating new members and fostering cohesiveness between newcomers and seasoned veterans. One way to

- Provide extra detail about the group structure and rules during facilitator introductions.
- Stress the importance of confidentiality and respect of others.
- Ask seasoned group members to introduce themselves first so that new members are socialized into the structure of the group.
- Pay extra attention to communicating a warm, inviting, nonjudgmental stance.
- Create an environment in which seasoned group members spontaneously provide support, encouragement, and information to new members.
- Identify similarities between continuing group members and newcomers.
- Remind the group that group members can have a range of treatment goals to relieve any anxiety about ambivalence toward abstinence.
- Relate new group members' experiences and problems to themes that have been discussed in previous groups and to the comprehensive cognitive model of addiction.
- Comment on the level of honesty and supportiveness between group members and explain that as people continue to attend, supportive relationships grow.
- Ask new members for input and feedback to ensure that they are benefiting from the group and are comfortable with the group format.

FIGURE 6.2. Strategies for integrating new members into the CTAG.

achieve these goals is for the facilitators to provide more detail about the group's structure and rules at the beginning of the session than they might if the session comprised only people who had attended at least one previous group. Although seasoned group members have heard this information many times, and new group members likely will have heard this in an individual meeting, such an explanation helps to focus the group on a common purpose. Issues to cover in an extended facilitator introduction of the group structure and rules include (1) the rationale for the heterogeneity of the group, (2) the interplay between psychoeducation and group discussion of cognitive and behavioral strategies, (3) the provision of authentic support to one another, (4) the structure of introductions and the manner in which the issues brought up in introductions determine the content of the group session, and (5) acceptance of group members who are at a variety of different stages of change. In addition, newcomers often feel most comfortable when they introduce themselves after the other group members have had a chance to share, as they will then have the opportunity to model their behavior after the more seasoned group members.

It is particularly important to discuss confidentiality when new members are present, which benefits both new members as well as existing members. Even in cases in which new members have had an individual meeting with a facilitator, they usually come to their first group session with a bit of trepidation. Common reasons for this trepidation are not knowing how much detail to disclose and wondering whether disclosing certain details will come back to haunt them. Similarly, existing group members need time to build trust with the new group member(s), so an explicit discussion of confidentiality assures existing group members that the standards of the group will be maintained. The facilitators may begin the discussion by asking questions such as "What must happen in this group to make it safe and productive for each of you?" or "Would those of you who have been here for a while describe the confidentiality rule and why it is important?" Some responses to these and similar questions might include "honesty," "openness," and "supportiveness." Group members are encouraged to discuss, in detail, the meaning of confidentiality and the potential consequences of violating confidentiality. At the end of this discussion, the facilitator makes a firm statement about the importance of confidentiality, such as "The most important rule in this group is that each of you honors each other's privacy and protect each other's confidentiality. Under no circumstances should anyone talk about another group member outside of the group because to do so would violate that person's trust in this group." The facilitators make it clear that group members will be asked to leave the group if it becomes evident that they have violated another member's confidentiality.

The following vignette demonstrates the smooth inclusion of a new group member. It logically follows from Brian's introduction, presented previously in this chapter:

FACILITATOR 1: We have one more introduction to complete before we move on to a focus on coping strategies. We are fortunate to have Rachel joining us today. Rachel, could you share a little bit about yourself regarding your addiction, the status of your addiction, your goals for your addiction, and other issues you might be dealing with at the moment?

RACHEL: (*shyly*) Hi, my name is Rachel. (*pauses, and some of the group members say, "Hi Rachel"*) I'm really nervous about the group, well, and nervous about everything going on in my life in general. Uh, my addiction is, um, that I drink too much. (*pauses again*)

FACILITATOR 1: It's a big step to be here, Rachel. And I think you're in the right place, as we've had many members who've struggled with drinking too much who have benefited a great deal from the group.

MICHAEL: I've been in the group for a long time, and drinking is probably the most common problem that group members bring to the table.

RACHEL: (*smiling gratefully at Michael*) Thanks.

FACILITATOR 2: Michael is absolutely right. Thanks for sharing that, Michael. What is the status of your drinking, and what is your ultimate goal?

RACHEL: (*clearing throat*) Well, I haven't had anything to drink for about a week now, since my family did one of those interventions. (Many group members give thumbs-up signals.) My family wants me to quit drinking altogether. I don't know, though.

FACILITATOR 1: (*gently*) So it sounds like you are still in the process of deciding upon the specific goal for your drinking?

RACHEL: (*sheepishly*) Yeah.

FACILITATOR 2: That's OK, Rachel. One thing you'll see about this group is that we respect a range of different goals for addictions. It is the goal of some group members to stay abstinent, but it is the goal of other group members to cut down whatever they are using or doing to a level that is no longer harmful for them.

RACHEL: (*looking more hopeful*) Really? I thought that most treatments for alcoholism say that you have to give it up completely.

ELLEN: Rachel, my addiction is overeating, but I can't give up eating completely. Obviously, we have to eat to survive. So I'm having to figure out how to modify my behavior.

RACHEL: Wow, this is all new to me. I'll have to think about this. My drinking really has only gotten bad over the past several months. Before that I was able to have a glass of wine or two at social occasions and stop there. I'd really like to go back to that. That's one of the reasons why I haven't joined AA—because I didn't think they'd understand.

FACILITATOR 1: The more you participate in the group, the more you'll be able to clarify your precise goals for your drinking. And the group will be there with you every step of the way as you work toward those goals. Are there any other issues you're struggling with?

RACHEL: Just getting my life back together. I really put my kids in danger a few times by driving them to their activities after drinking. So a lot of family members and close friends are really angry at me.

FACILITATOR 1: So, am I correct in sensing that you could resonate with the other members of the group who indicated that their addiction has caused problems in relationships with others?

RACHEL: Yes, definitely.

There are several aspects of this vignette that deserve note, as they represent specific ways that new group members can be integrated successfully into the ongoing group. First, Facilitator 1 mentioned that the group was "fortunate" to have Rachel join them. Use of language that communicates a warm, welcoming stance is inviting to the new group member and reassuring to existing group members. Second, Facilitator 1 sensed Rachel's apprehension during the introduction and expressed another encouraging statement, that she was taking a big step by trying out the group, and reassured her that alcohol use is a common issue discussed by many group members. Third, other group members chimed in to show support and communicate that their experiences resonated with hers. Facilitator 2 specifically reinforced Michael's observation with the intention of increasing the likelihood that other group members would interact directly with Rachel in a supportive manner as well. This comment also demonstrated to Rachel that there are similarities between the problems she is experiencing and problems experienced by other group members. Finally, when Facilitator 1 learned that Rachel was ambivalent about her specific goal for her drinking, Facilitator 2 took the opportunity to educate her (and remind the group) that a range of goals of group members is respected and that there is not one goal that fits all. Other strategies for integrating new members into the group include commenting explicitly on the level of trust and honesty in the group, showing the new member that supportive relationships will grow as they continue to attend sessions, and soliciting direct feedback from them to ensure that they believe they are benefiting from the group and are comfortable with the group format.

Despite their best intentions, facilitators sometimes find that the integration of a new group member does not run as smoothly as the previous vignette illustrates. In some instances, this occurs when something prohibits the new group member from fully engaging in the group, such as severe anxiety (which can lead to a lack of engagement), defensiveness (which can lead to behavior that is perceived as aggressive by other group members), or pronounced psychopathology (which can lead to a focus on the new group member at the expense of other group members and at the expense of the established "culture" of the group). In other instances, this occurs when existing group members are threatened by the new group member or have an adverse reaction to the material that the new group member is discussing. In fact, it is most common for difficulties integrating a new member into the group to result from a combination of these factors. Consider the following vignette:

FACILITATOR 1: We have one more introduction to complete before we move on to a focus on coping strategies. We are fortunate to have Jennifer joining us today. Jennifer, could you share a little bit about yourself regarding your addiction, the status of your addiction, your goals for your addiction, and other issues you might be dealing with at the moment?

JENNIFER: I have a lot of addictions—smoking, drinking, drugs, you name it. But I think the real issue is that I was repeatedly sexually abused by my grandfather all throughout my childhood, and that's why I am the way I am. He lived with us, and he came into my room every night and.... (*provides graphic details for several minutes, and some group members appear visibly uncomfortable*) So, if I can just talk about all of that and finally get that off of my chest, I think that my drinking and drug use will get better.

FACILITATOR 2: (*gently*) Jennifer, I'm very sorry to hear that your childhood was so difficult. Let me state the specific purpose of this group....

JENNIFER: (*cutting off Facilitator 2*) I just really need to talk about all of this, you know? Because....

FACILITATOR 2: It is certainly reasonable that you would want to get some help to address these experiences. In our experience, issues like this can be addressed in more than one way. This particular group focuses on addiction, and the one thing that links group members' experience is the fact that they are struggling or have struggled with addiction in the past. So, in *this* group, we'll be focusing on those issues that are shared by most, if not all, group members. However, another way for you to address your difficult childhood is to participate in individual psychotherapy so that a mental health professional can work with you, one-on-one, to give you the time you need to talk about these issues.

JENNIFER: I don't see why I can't talk about my childhood here, since all of my addictions stem from my grandfather's abuse.

FACILITATOR 1: I have an idea. Why don't you observe this group today to see whether this is right for you? When the group is over, you, Facilitator 2, and I can talk more to determine whether this is a good match for you. At that time, we can also give you a referral for individual psychotherapy so that you are sure to have a place where you can address these painful issues.

JENNIFER: (*pouting*) Well, OK. I just really need something quick. I've received all kinds of treatment, over and over, and nothing sticks. (*escalating*) I'm really desperate. I need people to listen to me. And....

FACILITATOR 1: I hear what you're saying, Jennifer. You have my word that we will spend some time with you after group to sort all of this out and get you all of the services that you need.

Although, technically, Jennifer was appropriate for the group because she struggled with addictive behavior, it quickly became clear that she had another agenda, in that she wanted to spend a great deal of time talking about her childhood sexual abuse. Her responses in session suggested that she was not responsive to subtle interventions to shape her behavior. The facilitators responded in a manner that communicated empathy about the difficulties with which she is currently struggling, but that also communicated an equally firm stance that the focus of the group is to be on addictions and their consequences. They made it clear to her that they are committed to helping her get the appropriate treatment, but that individualized attention for this purpose would have to take place outside of the group. Furthermore, their suggestion to "observe" the group communicated (1) that it was expected that her problems would not consume the majority of the group's attention, and (2) that it might be determined that the group is not the best match for her needs. Fortunately, Jennifer responded to this intervention, and her remaining contributions in that group session were small but appropriate. At the end of the session, Facilitator 1 met with Jennifer in his office to discuss her needs and make referrals, and Facilitator 2 took extra care to interact with each group member as he or she was leaving and monitor any lasting adverse effects of Jennifer's graphic references to her childhood sexual abuse.

Introductions When There Are No New Group Members

On occasion, facilitators observe that the CTAG's composition has been fairly static for a period of several weeks, such that the same members attend on a regular basis, and no new members are being integrated into the group. In these instances, facilitators can amend introductions to meet the group's needs and maximize the amount of time devoted to the cognitive and behavioral strategies. Some CTAG facilitators have used the concept of the "check-in," such that group members briefly mention the status of their addiction in the past week and other issues with which they are concerned. At times, the majority of the check-in can be devoted to a report on each member's implementation of the homework assignment that was developed in the previous session.

When facilitators amend the introduction process, they should take care to do so in collaboration with the group members, such that the group decides the topics to cover during introductions. Moreover, facilitators should never amend introductions in this manner when there is a new group member, a group member who has only attended a few sessions, or a group member who has been away for a period of time. For these individuals, the full introduction will help to orient (or reorient) them to the group, learn or be reminded of the names of fellow group members, and focus on goals. We also encourage facilitators to educate the group about the cognitive model in every session, no matter how redundant it seems, in order to reinforce the philosophy that underlies group interventions.

EDUCATION ABOUT THE COGNITIVE MODEL

During group member introductions, facilitators are vigilant to identify opportunities to educate the group about the cognitive approach to understanding addictions. At times, facilitators may educate about many aspects of the comprehensive cognitive model of addiction; at other times, they may only educate about the basics, such as the associations between triggers, cognition, and subsequent slips and lapses. Facilitators determine the amount of detail in light of the number of people attending that day's group, the number and severity of concerns discussed during introductions, and the number of new members and their attitude toward the group. For example, when only a small number of group members attend a session (e.g., 5 to 6 people), facilitators might take the opportunity to illustrate many components of the comprehensive cognitive model of addiction because introductions will take only a short period of time. In contrast, facilitators likely would not take this approach when a large number of group members are present (e.g., 12 or more people) because a larger chunk of the session might be devoted to introductions.

The presence of one or more new group members may also influence the amount of the comprehensive cognitive model of addiction is presented to group members. If there are many new group members, it would be logical to take extra time to describe the cognitive model so that they have a global understanding of the cognitive and behavioral factors that contribute to their addiction and the manner in which the group can address those factors. This approach can be especially useful when several of the new group members are enthusiastic about treatment and are actively seeking out information about their addiction. However, if several of those new group members are ambivalent about treatment, then extensive psychoeducation might be off-putting for them, and it might be more fruitful to focus on straightforward cognitive behavioral interventions in order to motivate them for change.

We realize that novice facilitators might be left with many questions about how to educate the group about the cognitive model in any one instance. We encourage facilitators to use the cognitive case conceptualization of the group as a whole (see Chapter 5) to guide their decision and to be sure that they can articulate a clear rationale for whatever choice they make. Although this might sound daunting to clinicians who are learning how to implement CTAGs, we view the flexibility of the CTAG as its strength, as facilitators can tailor each stand-alone session to the needs and stages of change of the group members in attendance. The key to making these decisions is that they (1) are guided by a sound rationale, rather than being made in a hasty or reactive manner; (2) follow from the case conceptualization of the group as a whole; and (3) implemented in as much a collaborative manner with the group members as is possible.

In the session from which the previous vignette was taken, it was clear that Ellen and Brian were having substantial difficulties in many areas of their lives. From previous experience, the facilitators knew that Ellen was willing to share her "story" with the group in most circumstances, with the view that she could be helpful to others, whereas Brian often became more depressed and, on occasion, even suicidal when his problems were highlighted to the group. Thus, the facilitators tentatively chose to focus on Ellen's addiction for the illustration of the cognitive model. They did not choose Michael because, as the longest-standing member of the group, Michael's addiction was often highlighted in other sessions. In addition, although Michael's 6-month-long abstinence was an inspiration to many, in this particular session, the facilitators hypothesized that highlighting his success would inadvertently facilitate a negative comparison with Brian, which would exacerbate Brian's depression. The facilitators did not choose Allison because she was new to the group, and they wanted to ensure that she was acclimated and comfortable before putting any spotlight on her. The facilitators also did not choose Dave, as Dave's tone of voice and mannerisms suggested that he is not completely invested in group and that he might not readily provide personal examples to illustrate the cognitive model.

Furthermore, the facilitators chose to share only the basics of the cognitive model for two reasons: (1) a more extensive discussion of the comprehensive cognitive model of addiction was presented the previous week, which was Allison's first meeting; and (2) it appeared that there was a common theme among group members' concerns that required much attention. The following is a example of the manner in which the facilitators illustrated the basic aspects of the cognitive model to the group, using Ellen's circumstances as an example. As she spoke, Facilitator 2 wrote the constructs on a whiteboard, much like the figures presented in Chapter 2, and drew arrows to demonstrate the associations among them:

FACILITATOR 1: Ellen, do you mind if we illustrate the cognitive model in light of some of the things that you're experiencing?

ELLEN: Sure, I'd be happy to do that. I've actually been thinking about those boxes and circles a lot to understand how I've gotten myself into such a rut.

FACILITATOR 1: According to the cognitive model of addiction, people are most likely to engage in addictive behaviors following certain triggers or cues. These triggers can be internal or external. Internal triggers include emotions like depression and loneliness, as well as physical sensations like withdrawal symptoms, pain, hunger, and fatigue. External triggers can include people, places, and things associated in some way with your addiction. Ellen, what do you think are the triggers that have been associated with your overeating lately?

ELLEN: Well, I think you really got it when you mentioned depression and loneliness.

FACILITATOR 2: (*writes "depression/loneliness" in a box labeled "trigger" on the whiteboard*)

ELLEN: Maybe an external trigger is seeing one of those commercials on TV. We just had the holidays; it was hard to watch all of those commercials with happy families sitting around the Christmas tree laughing and opening up presents.

FACILITATOR 1: What makes depression, loneliness, and TV commercials triggers?

ELLEN: I guess because I believe that the only way I can feel better is to eat something I like.

FACILITATOR 1: Exactly! (*turning to the entire group*) Triggers like these are powerful because they can activate addiction-related thoughts and beliefs. We call those thoughts and beliefs *cognitions*. According to the cognitive model of addiction, the most important difference between people with and without addictions is how they think. Triggers typically activate two types of thoughts—anticipatory and relief-oriented. Who remembers what those are?

ALLISON: I think I remember you saying that the anticipation ones focus on the good things associated with using, or smoking, or whatever, and that the relief ones focus on what the person is escaping.

FACILITATOR 1: You have a great memory, Allison. Ellen, what thoughts are getting activated in response to your depression and loneliness?

ELLEN: I don't know, I just get really upset.

FACILITATOR 1: You get really upset, but then somehow your mind goes to eating.

ELLEN: I guess I think that I can't bear this loneliness without eating.

FACILITATOR 1: So your cognition is relief-oriented. You don't believe you can handle these emotions if you don't eat.

ELLEN: Yes, I suppose you're right.

FACILITATOR 1: Once we have those anticipatory and relief-oriented thoughts, it's easy to give ourselves permission to engage in the addictive behavior. We call those thoughts facilitating thoughts. Ellen, do you have any facilitating thoughts?

ELLEN: It seems like I have those nonstop. It's like, no one wants me, I'm all alone, so what does it matter if I'm fat?

FACILITATOR 2: (writes Ellen's relief-oriented and facilitating thoughts in the appropriate boxes on the whiteboard and explains the manner in which these cognitions exacerbate urges and cravings and lead to addictive behavior)

FACILITATOR 1: We won't go into this in detail today so that we can start to address the issues that you all identified briefly in the introductions; however, can we take a minute for you all to remember some of the things that predispose us to addiction?

MICHAEL: We've talked a lot about childhood experiences.

FACILITATOR 1: Right, formative experiences that shape how we view the world and how we look at the addiction. Anything else?

BRIAN: Problems like depression and anger. Those can make addiction worse.

FACILITATOR 1: You got it. Anything else?

ALLISON: What I remember from last week is that even things like a person's personality can make them more likely to be an addict.

FACILITATOR : Great job. And why is it important to have an idea about these background factors?

ELLEN: They help us to understand why we developed a problem?

FACILITATOR 1: That's right. And they also give us additional pathways for making change. The more sessions you attend, the more you will address many parts of this model in the interest of recovering from your addiction. We'll certainly spend time working with the cognitions and behaviors that you experience when you are faced with a trigger. But we'll also focus on managing and overcoming the consequences of your addiction, like the relationship problems you have identified today. And, even more, we'll discuss some of the background factors that made you vulnerable to develop a problem with addictions and ways to curb some of those factors.

IDEAS FOR SESSION TOPICS

Although the *structure* of group is consistent across sessions (i.e., introductions, including a discussion of the cognitive model; cognitive and behavioral strategies; homework; closure), the *content* of the focus of discussion varies from session to session and depends on the concerns introduced by group members during introductions. In fact, this is another reason why it is helpful to have two facilitators, so that one facilitator can identify these commonalities while the other facilitator is leading the group. Facilitators should always be prepared with a range of topics that could assume focus in that session and be relevant to most, if not all, group members. For example, because each group member has struggled with at least one addictive behavior, work on relapse or on managing urges and cravings should almost always be relevant. In other instances, the group is split on their view of the most important concern on which to focus in group. In this case, facilitators can choose the topic that has been introduced most often across multiple sessions, not only in the current session. Facilitators can also solicit the group's agreement to focus on one topic in the current session, and then save the other topic for the subsequent session. In the vignettes presented earlier in this chapter, a clear theme emerged—relationship difficulties. With the group's agreement, they focused the majority of their time to consider cognitive and behavioral strategies for understanding and addressing relationship problems.

Figure 6.3 displays a list of common content areas addressed in CTAGs. It is important to acknowledge that the topics of CTAGs are in no way limited to this list—the group can address *any* topic as long as it is approached from a cognitive behavioral framework. We have supervised groups focused on unique topics such as symptoms of sexually transmitted diseases, typically observed gender differences in the handling of relationships, and children of group members who are exhibiting signs of addictive behavior. In the next several chapters of this volume, we demonstrate the range of cognitive and behavioral strategies that can serve as foci in individual CTAG sessions.

SUMMARY

Introductions serve a purpose that is much more complex than making sure group members know the names and addictions of other members. During introductions, themes that apply to many group members begin to emerge, and facilitators use that information to decide upon a topic for the coping skills component of the CTAG. Moreover, facilitators select one of the group member's problems to illustrate the cognitive model of addiction, and other

- Managing urges and cravings
- Dealing with slips, lapses, and relapse
- Managing mood disturbance (e.g., depression, anxiety, anger)
- Coping with the rules and structure of supervised living
- Developing new interests and pastimes
- Repairing damaged relationships
- Developing new relationships
- Complying with other psychiatric, addiction, medication, and social service interventions
- Coping with the medical consequences of addictive behavior
- Coping with the financial consequences of addictive behavior
- Dealing with the aftermath of the legal consequences of addictive behavior
- Managing impulsivity and the inability to delay reward
- Developing self-care strategies

FIGURE 6.3. Common content areas addressed in CTAGs.

group members are encouraged to contribute to identifying pieces of the model and generalizing it to their own addictive behaviors. During introductions, group cohesiveness starts to develop. In addition, group members learn that others are struggling with similar issues but that success is possible, thereby attaining a sense of universality and building hope. Thus, introductions are crucial in fostering many of Yalom and Leszcz's (2005) therapeutic factors and in setting the stage for the cognitive and behavioral work that will be done during the rest of the session.

FORM 6.1. CTAG Attendance and Summary Form

Group Member's Name	Addictions (Past and Present)	Status of Addictive Behaviors	Goals (e.g., Abstinence, Reduction)	Other Issues
Member 1 _____				
Member 2 _____				
Member 3 _____				
Member 4 _____				
Member 5 _____				
Member 6 _____				

(cont.)

Group Member's Name	Addictions (Past and Present)	Status of Addictive Behaviors	Goals (e.g., Abstinence, Reduction)	Other Issues
Member 7 _____				
Member 8 _____				
Member 9 _____				
Member 10 _____				
Member 11 _____				
Member 12 _____				

CHAPTER 7 | Evaluating Thoughts and Beliefs

According to the cognitive model, the cognitions that we experience are strongly associated with our subsequent emotional reactions and behavioral responses. If these cognitions are inaccurate or unhelpful, than we are at risk of reacting in a way that increases our emotional distress and/ or is self-defeating. One important activity in cognitive therapy is to help patients become aware of these cognitions, develop skills to evaluate the degree to which they are accurate and helpful, and if it is concluded that they are not accurate and/or helpful, then to modify them so that they are more balanced.

As described in Chapter 2, there are two levels of cognition to consider in understanding our emotional reactions and behavioral responses. *Situational cognitions* are the thoughts, images, and outcome expectancies that are activated in any one circumstance. Some of these cognitions pertain to the engagement in addictive behaviors, such as anticipatory outcome expectancies (e.g., "It will feel good to get high"), relief-oriented expectancies (e.g., "I just need to escape"), and facilitating thoughts (e.g., "I deserve this because I've been through a lot lately"). Other situational cognitions represent automatic thoughts that are, more generally, related to emotional experiences. For example, if a person has to speak in front of a group of people, he or she might have the automatic thought, "I will screw up," and subsequently experience nervousness. If a person receives a low grade on an important exam, he or she might have the automatic thought, "I'm not smart enough for this class," and subsequently experience dejection. Situational cognitions can also take the form of mental images, such as visions of "worst-case scenarios" for the future or memories of aversive events we have experienced in the past. The common features among all of these cognitions are that (1) they are activated by external or internal triggers, (2) they affect our mood and subsequent behavioral reactions, and (3) with practice, they can be "caught" and evaluated before they cause damage.

Over time, CTAG facilitators see a pattern to the typical situational cognitions that particular group members report. These patterns point to *underlying beliefs* that drive the cognitions that are experienced in any one circumstance. As mentioned in Chapters 2 and 5, there are two kinds of underlying beliefs that are important in conceptualizing any one group member's cognitive profile—basic beliefs about oneself, the world, and/or the future, and addiction-related beliefs. Basic beliefs and addiction-related beliefs often are not readily recognized by group members, at least when they first begin to participate in sessions. However, with practice in applying the strategies to identify, evaluate, and modify situational cognitions, group members begin to recognize their underlying beliefs and apply strategies for evaluating and modifying them, as well. Although great change can be seen when group members modify inaccurate and unhelpful situational cognitions, the most substantial change usually occurs when unhelpful underlying beliefs are addressed.

Consider the case of Michael. In Chapter 5, we learned that he received messages from his father and his brother that he was not "manly" enough because he did not spend time with them doing the activities that they found meaningful, such as working with them in the garage. Over time, he developed the idea that he is "an incompetent man," which is an example of an unhelpful basic belief about himself. In one CTAG session, Michael indicated that he made a small mistake on a job he was doing for his law firm. After some questioning, he recognized that he experienced the automatic thoughts, "I'm stupid" and "I'm such a loser" after he learned of the mistake. If Michael had not had the core belief that he is an incompetent man, he might have experienced a more balanced thought such as "It's too bad I made that mistake" or "I'll have to watch out not to make the same mistake twice." Instead, Michael had the self-deprecating automatic thoughts of being stupid and a loser because the situation easily activated his basic belief that he is an incompetent man. It is not surprising that he became quite down after this incident, making him vulnerable to a slip or a lapse. This chapter outlines several strategies that facilitators can help group members to acquire in identifying, evaluating, and modifying situational cognitions and underlying beliefs. In the language of the TTM (Prochaska & DiClemente, 2005), these strategies achieve counterconditioning because group members acquire the skills to replace problematic cognitions with healthier cognitions.

WORKING WITH SITUATIONAL COGNITIONS

Because automatic thoughts occur so quickly, many people do not real-ize that they have been activated or that they are having a palpable effect on their mood. The same is true for outcome expectancies—they are so practiced that patients with addictions take them as fact and do not ques-tion them. The following section describes the first step in helping group members to evaluate their situational cognitions, which involves developing strategies for slowing down and identifying these cognitions. The subse-quent parts of this section describe strategies for evaluating and responding to these cognitions.

Identifying Situational Cognitions

Figure 7.1 summarizes some common questions that can be asked to iden-tify situational cognitions. Some of the questions in this exhibit are ques-tions that are generally used by cognitive therapists who treat a range of conditions; other questions are specific to situational cognitions that might be experienced when group members are faced with a trigger to engage in addictive behavior. It is common to hear facilitators asking these questions of group members when they are engaging in the process of identifying and modifying inaccurate and unhelpful cognitions. However, facilitators also aim for group members to begin to ask these questions of themselves, so that they can "catch" these situational cognitions when they are experienc-ing them in the moment. Thus, facilitators model the use of these questions in session, and they also help group members brainstorm ways to identify these cognitions on their own. In other words, group members acquire skill and practice in asking these questions of themselves when they notice an urge, a craving, or a negative change in their mood.

The most straightforward way to elicit situational cognitions is to ask the question, "What was running through your mind in that situation?" Facilitators will quickly see that there is a broad range in the degree to which group members are able to answer this question accurately. For some group members, the cognitive model resonates well with the manner in which they typically approach their life, and they are easily able to identify unhelpful automatic thoughts and outcome expectancies that disrupt their mood and increase the likelihood of engaging in addictive behavior. How-ever, other group members have great difficulty identifying these cogni-tions. In these instances, it is useful for facilitators to help group members to estimate the thoughts that they might have been thinking, such as by asking them to guess what was running through their mind or to speculate about the thoughts that might run through the mind of someone similar. If

- What was running through your mind in that situation?
- What would you guess was running through your mind in that situation?
- If a similar person were in that situation, what might run through his or her mind?
- Would you have been thinking _____ or _____ ? (*Facilitator provides a couple of plausible possibilities.*)
- Were you imagining something that might happen or remembering something that happened?
- What did this situation mean to you or say about you?
- Were you thinking _____ ? (*Facilitator provides a cognition opposite to the expected response.*)
- To assess anticipatory outcome expectancies: Were you thinking about how good it would feel to [insert name of addiction]? What specifically were you focused on?
- To assess relief-oriented outcome expectancies: Were you hoping that [insert name of addiction] would help you to avoid or escape something uncomfortable? What specifically were you focused on?
- To assess facilitating thoughts: How did you give yourself permission to [insert name of addiction]?
- To assess self-efficacy: What do you say to yourself about your ability to cope?

FIGURE 7.1. Questions to elicit situational cognitions. Many of these questions are found in J. S. Beck (2011).

group members continue to experience difficulty eliciting situational cognitions using these strategies, facilitators can be even more directive, such as by providing group members with two plausible situational cognitions and asking them to choose one. Facilitators can also ask targeted questions that get at anticipatory outcome expectancies, relief-oriented outcome expectancies, facilitating thoughts, and thoughts related to self-efficacy, which are presented at the bottom of Figure 7.1.

The following is a vignette that describes the ebb and flow of eliciting situational cognitions in a CTAG session. Notice that group members do not necessarily identify the most relevant thought on the first attempt—sometimes they report descriptions of what was going on in the situation rather than what the situation meant to them; other times, they report emotions instead of thoughts. It is the job of the facilitators to patiently guide group members through the process and gently educate them about the distinction between thoughts and emotions. It is an ongoing process to model the cognitive therapy approach to group members, and group members often learn strategies from one another as the exercise progresses:

FACILITATOR 1: Dave, you mentioned that you had a slip over the weekend—you got drunk and also smoked two joints. Tell us about what was going on that led up to that.

DAVE: It was just a bad day. My girlfriend told me that she thinks she's pregnant. It was just way too much; I had to get out of the house.

MICHAEL: Oh, wow. I can imagine that was tough.

FACILITATOR 1: I agree, that sounds really heavy. When your girlfriend told you she thought she was pregnant—what was running through your mind just then?

DAVE: Panic.

FACILITATOR 1: OK, panic. Is panic a thought, or is it a feeling?

DAVE: It's both, because I was scared shitless, and I thought to myself, "Panic!"

FACILITATOR 1: I hear what you are saying, that perhaps "panic" was the first thing that came to mind. However, I'm wondering what underlies that idea of "panic!" What did it mean to you that your girlfriend told you she was pregnant?

DAVE: I don't know.... I mean, it's the last thing I need right now. I don't even know if I want to stay with her. All we do right now is fight. And a baby is just going to be more stressful, lots more money, crying all the time.... (*shaking head*)

FACILITATOR 2: It sounds like you're anticipating a lot of negative consequences if she really ends up being pregnant. What does that mean for you, for your life?

DAVE: (*long pause*) I'm stuck. I'm never going to get out of this situation.

FACILITATOR 2: You hit the nail on the head—that's a logical thought that is associated with the panic reaction. In fact, it's natural for anyone to have the emotional reaction of panic when they believe they are trapped in an undesirable situation. Has anyone else experienced similar types of thoughts?

ALLISON: Dave, one time I remember the same reaction when I thought I couldn't get the money together to go back to school. I thought I'd be stuck in my crummy cashier job forever. I just about had a panic attack.

In this example, the facilitators chose to guide Dave in identifying the verbal meaning that the situation had for him. However, Dave's description also suggested that he was experiencing powerful and distressing mental imagery. The facilitators could have chosen to elicit Dave's mental images instead:

> DAVE: I don't know.... I mean, it's the last thing I need right now. I don't even know if I want to stay with her. All we do right now is fight. And a baby is just going to be more stressful, lots more money, crying all the time.... (*shaking head*)
>
> FACILITATOR 1: Dave, it sounds like you are imagining what it would be like for the baby to be born. Describe what you see.
>
> DAVE: (*visibly shaken*) I see us still living in our God-forsaken cramped trailer, but now the baby is making it even more cramped. The baby is screaming constantly, and neither of us can get any sleep. Dishes are piled up because the baby takes up so much time that my girlfriend doesn't have time to do anything else around the house. And I'm like an old man—worn out, can't go out and have any fun, maybe even having to work two jobs to make ends meet.

This vignette illustrates the general process of identifying situational cognitions. However, CTAG facilitators usually need to take the exercise one step further than many other cognitive therapists—not only must they work with group members to identify automatic thoughts that are associated with emotional distress in particular situations, but they also must work with group members to examine the outcome expectancies and facilitating thoughts that are subsequently activated and the manner in which these cognitions influence behavior. The identification of these addiction-related thoughts will help group members understand the manner in which difficult situations and even thoughts about difficult situations can serve as triggers for urges to engage in addictive behavior. It also helps group members to understand the manner in which facilitating thoughts are activated and increase the likelihood that patients will slip.

> FACILITATOR 1: So it sounds like you had a really tough conversation that brought up a lot of negative thoughts and images for you. What happened after that?
>
> DAVE: I tried to sit down and numb my mind with a race on TV, but it wasn't working. I had to get out of there.
>
> FACILITATOR 2: Is that when you went to the bar where you used to hang out?
>
> DAVE: Yeah.
>
> FACILITATOR 2: When you were sitting and watching TV, when it

wasn't helping you to relax, what was running through your mind then?

DAVE: I have to get out of here.

FACILITATOR 2: OK, that makes sense. How did you get from there to the bar?

DAVE: I was just like, "Screw it. I might as well go get drunk because I'm not going to have any fun in about 7 months."

FACILITATOR 2: A-hah. So you had a thought related to your substance use. Dave, what was the trigger in this situation?

DAVE: Being pissed off.

ELLEN: And, also Dave, it seemed like you were feeling really wound up, unsettled. And like you didn't know how to calm yourself down.

DAVE: Yeah, that was it, too, I guess.

FACILITATOR 2: So you were experiencing a range of intense emotions, and the way you chose to cope with them, watching a race on TV, wasn't effective. And then you had the thought, "Screw it. I might as well go get drunk because I'm not going to have any fun in about 7 months." What kind of thought is that?

DAVE: I don't know. The only thing I could do at the time.

(*Both facilitators look around the room to other group members.*)

BRIAN: A facilitating thought?

FACILITATOR 1: You got it. And what's the effect of the facilitating thought when it comes to mind?

DAVE: I guess it made it easier for me to just go out to the bar instead of try to think of another way to deal with the situation.

One standard cognitive therapy tool for helping patients respond to automatic thoughts is the Thought Record. The Four-Column Thought Record (see Form 7.1 at the end of the chapter) is a worksheet that allows group members to record situations or triggers, situational cognitions, emotions, and subsequent behavioral responses. Many standard cognitive therapy texts suggest having patients initially focus on identifying situations, thoughts, and emotions in the format of a Three-Column Thought Record (cf. A. T. Beck, Rush, Shaw, & Emery, 1979; Greenberger & Padesky, 1995). We have expanded that Thought Record to one that is four columns so that group members can observe the manner in which situational cognitions and related emotional experiences fuel behavioral outcomes, especially the engagement in addictive behavior. Repeated use of the Four-Column

Thought Record reinforces the strong association among situational cognitions, emotions, and behavioral responses, and demonstrates that there are many points of intervention to "break the cycle" of engaging in addictive or otherwise self-defeating behavior.

Facilitators should have Four-Column Thought Records available if they judge that they would be useful to complete during the course of a session. Advantages to completing Four-Column Thought Records in session are (1) group members will have a concrete and personal example of the process by which they can identify situational cognitions in their daily lives, and (2) the act of writing helps to solidify the steps of the process. However, in some instances, facilitators judge that it is cumbersome to complete Four-Column Thought Records in session. Group members may have differing levels of ability and willingness to complete worksheets. Whereas some members might easily grasp the concepts in the Four-Column Thought Record and complete it quickly in session, others might struggle. Facilitators must monitor the ease with which group members complete Four-Column Thought Records, assist those who are having difficulty, and simultaneously acknowledge and validate those who have finished the exercise. One strategy for managing patients with varying skill levels is to pair experienced group members with inexperienced group members and to have them complete the Four-Column Thought Records together.

Regardless of whether facilitators choose to use Four-Column Thought Records in session or simply identify group members' situational cognitions through questioning, they should take care to work with group members to identify ways in which this exercise can be used in their daily lives outside of the group session. The following vignette occurred toward the end of the group session, when Dave and other group members had identified powerful situational cognitions that increased their urges and cravings:

FACILITATOR 1: You all have worked very hard today. Each of you identified situational thoughts that either exacerbated your urges and cravings or made you feel sad and uncomfortable. Can each of you tell me how this exercise is going to make a difference for you?

MICHAEL: Since I've been in the group for awhile, I've done this before. I can tell you that it makes a big difference in my life. Those facilitating thoughts come up so quickly that, if I'm not careful, the next thing you know, I'm in a compromising situation.

BRIAN: Yeah, I know that my thinking about gambling—hell, my life in general—is messed up. But I'm not sure what to do about it.

FACILITATOR 2: I'm glad you mentioned that, Brian. We spent a large chunk of today on identifying the thoughts and images that come up in certain situations, especially when we are triggered. But that's only the first step. As a group, we can think about ways to actually deal with those thoughts and images. In the future, would you be up for that?

BRIAN: Yeah, definitely.

ALLISON: I'd be up for that, too. I know that I'm playing with fire when I tell myself it's OK to have even just one cigarette.

FACILITATOR 1: Great. The first step in this process is recognizing when these kinds of thoughts pop into our minds. Would you all be willing to track these thoughts in between now and our next session?

ELLEN: I sure would.

FACILITATOR 1: *(catching Dave's eye as he is looking around the room)*

DAVE: I don't know, I doubt it. I mean, what's the point?

FACILITATOR 1: A critical question, Dave. *(turning to the group)* You'll only be motivated to use what you learn in treatment if you think there is a good reason behind it. What is the purpose of paying attention to your thoughts?

ELLEN: Because what we're thinking has a big effect on what we're feeling and on our behavior?

FACILITATOR 2: Exactly. So what happens if something you are thinking or saying to yourself isn't entirely accurate or helpful?

BRIAN: If it's something bad, then it can just make us feel worse.

ALLISON: Yeah, and I guess it also just keeps that cycle of addiction going.

FACILITATOR 2: You're right. When we're stressed or in a difficult place in life, it's easy to have tunnel vision and focus on the negative, which just makes you feel worse. And when you're faced with the trigger, it's easy to focus on all of the reasons for engaging in addictive behavior, ignoring the consequences.

FACILITATOR 1: Dave, do you buy this idea? That your thinking plays a large role in affecting how you're feeling and whether you drink or smoke weed?

DAVE: I don't know, I don't even really think that I think about it. I just do it.

FACILITATOR 1: Many people, when they are first starting the group, say the same thing. Did any of the rest of you have a similar experience when you joined the group?

MICHAEL: I hear you, Dave. When I first joined the group, I thought it was kind of crazy, like mind over matter. I wasn't sure this was for me.

DAVE: So what changed?

MICHAEL: I just tried to keep an open mind. And practice too. I knew it was either this or I'd lose my family.

BRIAN: I think I'm still kind of doing what Dave said. I've been in and out of this group for a couple of years now, but I'm not really sure that I can figure out my thoughts when it counts. I don't mean to be discouraging, Dave, but it can take some time to get this.

FACILITATOR 1: That's why we call many of these thoughts automatic thoughts—because they come up so quickly that we don't even realize that we're experiencing them. And to me, that's all the more reason to start paying attention to them, so that you can slow down and recognize when they're getting you in trouble. Does that make sense to you?

DAVE: Yeah, I guess.

FACILITATOR 1: So would you be willing to pay attention to these thoughts in between our sessions so that, next time, we can start to figure out some ways to deal with them?

DAVE: If I remember.

FACILITATOR 2: Another good point. You have to remember to do this. How can you take what we're talking about in today's session and make sure you use it outside of session?

ALLISON: I think I'll keep a piece of paper in my purse, so that I can write down these thoughts when I notice them. I almost always have my purse with me.

ELLEN: I don't usually go anywhere, so I just keep a notepad on my end table, next to where I sit when I watch TV.

MICHAEL: I use my BlackBerry.

BRIAN: Yeah, I guess I can use my smartphone, too.

FACILITATOR 1: Dave, what about you? Do any of these ideas ring true with you?

DAVE: I don't have a smartphone. And I don't like to write things down, it reminds me too much of school.

BRIAN: I was like that too, the last time I came to this group on a regular basis. I didn't want to write anything down. (*pausing*) And look what happened. (*Group members give looks of sympathy.*) Even if your phone isn't a smartphone, can it do voice recordings?

DAVE: (*Doesn't know, so he hands phone to Brian, who figures out that his phone has this capability.*) OK, I guess recording these thoughts is better than having to write them down.

FACILITATOR 1: Great, thanks for helping Dave figure that out, Brian. This is an excellent example of the fact that everyone might use cognitive therapy in slightly different ways, but that you will all achieve the same goal—to identify the thoughts that get you into trouble, either with your addiction or with your mood.

FACILITATOR 2: And when you notice an urge, a craving, or a negative shift in mood, what do you ask yourself?

ELLEN: What was running through my mind at that moment?

FACILITATOR 2: Exactly. What was running through your mind.

This vignette demonstrates many important points for facilitators to keep in mind. First, Facilitator 1 asked group members how identifying situational cognitions will make a difference in their lives. Not only did this question evoke testimonials from seasoned group members about the power of this exercise, but it also allowed the facilitators to see that not everyone was on board with it. It is critical for group members to understand the rationale behind cognitive therapy strategies, buy into the possibility that the strategies will be helpful for them, and commit to practicing the strategies in between sessions (see Chapter 9 for a more detailed discussion of homework). Second, Facilitator 2 anticipated that future group sessions could be devoted to developing strategies to cope with the thoughts. Such a statement reassures group members that they are expected to get relief from their situational cognitions. Third, Facilitator 1 seized an opportunity to build group cohesiveness in light of Dave's apprehension about monitoring thoughts by identifying instances in which others had similar reactions. Fourth, this vignette shows that creativity plays an important role in the CTAG, as each group member can adapt the strategies according to his or her personal style and available resources. We encourage facilitators not to be tied to any one specific cognitive therapy technique, but instead to keep the fundamental goals and principles of cognitive therapy in mind as they creatively work with group members to devise individualized ways of implementing them. Finally, Facilitator 2 reinforced a crucial component of this exercise at the end of the vignette—reminding group members to ask themselves what was running through their minds.

Evaluating Situational Cognitions

Identifying situational cognitions is only half the battle. As members attend more and more sessions, they will be exposed to an array of strategies to take a step back and evaluate the situational cognitions that they identify. For some group members, this process is relatively straightforward, but for many group members, this process is a struggle and requires several weeks of diligent practice. It is usually helpful to develop homework assignments (see Chapter 9) so that group members can begin to apply the skills to evaluate situational cognitions in their daily lives.

Common Cognitive Distortions

Facilitators often find it useful to educate CTAG members about common cognitive distortions that characterize the nature of their situational cognitions (see Figure 7.2). By being exposed to these erroneous patterns of thinking, group members can "catch" themselves when they fall into predictable "traps." It is helpful for facilitators to be very familiar with this material in order to guide group members in identifying instances in which they fall into these traps as they participate in the session. The following vignette might have occurred when Dave was discussing his reaction to the news that his girlfriend might be pregnant:

> DAVE: I was just like, "Screw it. I might as well go get drunk because I'm not going to have any fun in about 7 months."

> FACILITATOR 2: (*to the group*) What kinds of cognitive distortions are evident in Dave's statement?

> ELLEN: Catastrophizing? Because you're not considering the fact that you might really fall in love with the baby.

> ALLISON: I don't know what a cognitive distortion is, but I think you could be catastrophizing because you don't even know for sure that your girlfriend is pregnant.

> FACILITATOR 2: What do you think, Dave?

> DAVE: Well, yeah, I know it's not for sure, but every day that passes, it's more and more likely that it's true.

> FACILITATOR 1: Any other cognitive distortions?

> MICHAEL: I would say that the thought, "I'm never going to have fun again" is all-or-nothing thinking. I mean, yes, when you have a baby, you have a lot less time to yourself. But that doesn't mean that you can *never* get a babysitter and do something that's fun. And as children grow up, they are more and more independent.

> DAVE: Yeah, yeah, I know all of that. But right now it doesn't sink in. All I can do is see myself being miserable.

1. **All-or-nothing thinking:** You view a situation in only two categories instead of a continuum.

2. **Catastrophizing:** You make a negative prediction about the future without considering other, more likely outcomes.

3. **Disqualifying the positive:** You unreasonably tell yourself that positive experiences, deeds, or qualities do not count.

4. **Emotional reasoning:** You think something might be true because you "feel" it so strongly, discounting evidence to the contrary.

5. **Labeling:** You put a fixed, global label on yourself or others without considering that the evidence might more reasonably lead to a less disastrous conclusion.

6. **Magnification/minimization:** When you evaluate yourself, another person, or a situation, you unreasonably magnify the negative and/or minimize the positive.

7. **Mental filter:** You pay undue attention to one negative detail instead of seeing the big picture.

8. **Mind reading:** You believe you know what others are thinking, failing to consider more likely possibilities.

9. **Overgeneralization:** You make a sweeping negative conclusion that goes far beyond the current situation.

10. **Personalization:** You believe others are behaving negatively because of you, without considering more plausible explanations for their behavior.

11. **"Should" and "must" statements:** You have a precise, fixed idea of how you and others should behave, and you overestimate how bad it is that these expectations are not met.

12. **Tunnel vision:** You see only the negative aspects of a situation.

FIGURE 7.2. Common cognitive distortions.

Adapted from J. S. Beck (2011). Copyright 2011 by Judith S. Beck. Reprinted in *Group Cognitive Therapy for Addictions* by Amy Wenzel, Bruce S. Liese, Aaron T. Beck, and Dara G. Friedman-Wheeler (Guilford Press, 2012). Permission to photocopy this figure is granted to purchasers of this book for personal use only (see copyright page for details). Purchasers may download a larger version of this figure from the book's page on The Guilford Press website.

FACILITATOR 1: Ah, an example of emotional reasoning. You *feel* a lot of negative emotions *right now*—anger, anxiety, apprehension— and so you're deciding that it will be horrible.

BRIAN: Maybe that's emotional reasoning, but trust me, Dave, if I were in this situation, I'd be having the exact same reaction you're having.

When facilitators notice that many group members are making statements consistent with the cognitive distortions listed in Figure 7.2, it is often helpful to take that opportunity to educate group members about cognitive distortions. The figure can easily be turned into a handout for group members. Many CTAG facilitators have given such a handout to group members, asked them to glance over it, and identify whether any of the cognitive distortions are particularly fitting for them. Over time, group members become familiar with this material and can recognize, on their own, when their automatic thoughts represent one or more cognitive distortions. Consider the following vignette, when the facilitators decided to take the opportunity to educate the group about cognitive distortions:

FACILITATOR 1: (*to the group as a whole*) Take a look at this list and tell me what jumps out at you as being characteristic of your thinking.

BRIAN: (*sighing*) I think they *all* apply to me. I'm a mess.

ELLEN: Sometimes I think I'm a mess, too, when I look at these sheets. But, Brian, you're taking a big step by coming back to group.

BRIAN: (*giving Ellen a weak smile*)

FACILITATOR 1: Actually, Brian, you're not the first person to say that. In fact, many people have that same observation—that most, if not all, of the cognitive distortions characterize their thinking. (*pausing so that Brian can see many group members nodding their heads*) One reason for this is that most people fall into these traps in way or another, even if they aren't having trouble with addictions. The problem is, when you're dealing with an addiction, falling into one of these traps could lead to a slip or a lapse.

MICHAEL: All-or-nothing thinking really applied to me when I first started a group. I used to look at life as either exciting or boring— and the only way to get excitement was to be living on the edge, either going to strip clubs or having some sort of relationship I couldn't have. Now, maybe life isn't as exciting as it used to be, but I'm able to see that it isn't boring either. Life is good in a different way. There is a lot of satisfaction with coming home to your wife and kids at the end of the day.

ALLISON: What's overgeneralization? I don't get it.

FACILITATOR 2: Can anyone help her out?

BRIAN: I think I'm doing it right now. I'm beating myself up over my recent slip, and I'm thinking that life will never get any better. That I have nothing going for me.

FACILITATOR 2: That's right on target, Brian. Overgeneralization is taking one incident or one detail, and assuming that that incident has implications for all areas of your life.

(*Group proceeds to identify examples of the remaining cognitive distortions.*)

FACILITATOR 1: So why is it important to recognize these cognitive distortions?

ELLEN: It's a quick way for me to stop my negative thinking. I say, there I go again, I'm personalizing, or I'm disqualifying the positive. I might not know how to think differently all the time, but at least I can recognize when I'm going down a road that will just leave me feeling sad and alone. (*pausing*) Brian, maybe looking at it like that would be helpful for you?

BRIAN: Yeah, maybe it would. Just putting on the brakes could help me feel better.

Examining the Validity of Situational Cognitions

A central goal of cognitive therapy is for patients to acquire the skills to evaluate the validity of inaccurate or unhelpful situational cognitions as they arise in the moment. The idea is not necessarily to disconfirm or invalidate the situational cognition; in fact, in many instances there is a "grain of truth" inherent in patients' cognitions. Instead, the questions described in this section can be used as a vehicle for group members to view their situational cognitions from a broader perspective than they might have otherwise, evaluating all of the pertinent evidence that supports and refutes these cognitions. By using these strategies, group members are able to appraise situations in a more balanced manner, taking into account all relevant information and evaluating it systematically.

Figure 7.3 lists common questions that can be asked in evaluating the validity of situational cognitions. During CTAG sessions, facilitators and group members can ask these questions as group members are grappling with their situational cognitions, and the figure can be turned into

- What evidence supports this idea? What evidence refutes this idea? On the basis of this evidence, what is the most logical conclusion?

- What's the worst that can happen? What's the best that can happen? What's the most realistic thing that can happen?

- Am I 100% sure of these awful consequences?

- What is the likelihood that _____ will occur?

- If _____ occurs, how bad, realistically, will that be?

- Does _____ equal or lead to _____ ?

- Is _____ really so consequential?

- Does _____ 's opinion reflect the opinion of others?

- What are some other explanations?

- What is the effect of believing this thought right now?

- Is it really useful for me to be focusing on this thought right now?

- Is this way of thinking worth it? Is this behavior worth it?

- What would I tell a friend who is in this situation?

- If I must be in this situation, what wisdom or insight can I gain from it?

- What are the short-term consequences of this behavior? The long-term consequences? Do the short-term consequences outweigh the long-term consequences?

- Will [insert name of addiction] truly improve my life?

FIGURE 7.3. Evaluating the validity of situational cognitions. Many of these questions are found in J. S. Beck (2011).

a handout for group members. The following vignette illustrates this process:

FACILITATOR 1: Dave, you had the idea "I might as well go get drunk because I'm not going to have any fun in about 7 months." How do you know that?

DAVE: Oh believe me, I know that. My girlfriend has a lot of trouble dealing with stress. She falls apart even when she has to deal with little things, like not getting the shift she wants at work. And I'm left to pick up the pieces. I guarantee you that I will be left to do all the work—holding down a job, paying the bills, probably even making dinner and cleaning the house.

FACILITATOR 2: Could some of you pitch in to help Dave take a good, hard look at the accuracy of this thought?

ELLEN: Well, have there been any other times when you and your girlfriend have had to face a lot of stress, where everything was turned upside down?

DAVE: Well, yeah, I guess last year when her mother was really sick. She was constantly running to her mother's place to take care of her, and it got worse and worse as her mom went downhill. And then when her mom actually died ... that was a tough time.

ALLISON: Ugh, I went through that a few years ago when my mom died.

FACILITATOR 2: That does sound really tough. And during that time, how were you affected?

DAVE: I guess she got even more irritable. I felt like I couldn't do anything right. So life at home was pretty miserable.

BRIAN: Did you really have to do *everything*, like you expected?

DAVE: Well, I had to do more because she wasn't there.

BRIAN: But was it *everything*?

DAVE: (*sighing*) No, I didn't have to do *everything*. Sometimes she would actually come home and make everything spotless because she said it took her mind off of the fact that her mother was dying.

FACILITATOR 1: So it sounds like, in this major time of stress, you did have to assume some extra responsibilities, but you didn't have to assume all responsibilities 100% of the time. Am I correct?

DAVE: Yeah, I guess when you put it that way.

MICHAEL: Yeah, this is good stuff. So how come you think this time will be different?

DAVE: (*frowning*) I don't know.

FACILITATOR 1: What might be a more balanced way of viewing this situation?

DAVE: (*begrudgingly*) I suppose that I have to accept that I will have more responsibility, but that I shouldn't just assume that I'll have to do *everything*.

FACILITATOR 1: This is a terrific example of getting some distance or perspective on our thoughts. For those of you who have been participating in the group for awhile, what are some other questions you ask yourself when you are anticipating awful consequences, like having to take on all of the major household responsibilities and not having any fun?

MICHAEL: Am I 100% sure of these consequences?

ELLEN: Does the fact that your girlfriend has a baby have to lead to never having fun?

BRIAN: And how useful is it for you to be dwelling on this, when you don't even know for sure that she is pregnant?

FACILITATOR 2: Those are great examples. Dave, how would you respond to those questions?

DAVE: (*a little sarcastically*) *No*, I guess I'm not 100% sure that stuff will happen.

FACILITATOR 1: Dave, I'm sensing a little bit of sarcasm. What's running through your mind right now?

DAVE: I guess I just don't buy it. I still think life is going to suck if she is pregnant. I don't think I can stop thinking about it. (*laughing sarcastically*) And I know I should just have her take a test. But I'm scared shitless to do it, because what if it says she's pregnant?

This example illustrates the fact that even when applied skillfully, the cognitive therapy process does not always result in a modification of inaccurate or unhelpful situational cognitions as planned. Often, group members require some practice with the approach in order to ensure that they are focusing on the *most* relevant situational cognitions that are associated with distress and that they are asking the *most* relevant questions to evaluate the cognition. In Dave's case, there are additional possibilities that might explain why the process of evaluating situational cognitions did not lead to a more balanced appraisal of the situation. For example, his statement "I guess I just don't buy it" raises the possibility that he has not fully invested in the cognitive approach. To address this possibility, the facilitators might take time to invite group members to assist him in reviewing the main tenets of the cognitive approach and to provide examples from their own lives in which the cognitive approach was relevant and useful. Another common obstacle is that patients understand "intellectually" that their situational cognition is distorted but do not believe it "emotionally" (J. S. Beck, 2011). In these cases, it is useful to focus on the "worst-case scenario" and realistically assess how bad that situation will be.

With practice, group members learn to ask questions of themselves in order to critically evaluate the accuracy and usefulness of their cognitions. In addition to evaluating the validity of situational cognitions related to general distress, it also is important for facilitators to help group members practice applying these strategies to the evaluation of outcome expectancies and facilitating thoughts that are activated in response to triggers. The following vignette illustrates a successful intervention with Ellen regarding her overeating:

ELLEN: *(tearfully)* Instead of sticking with my new weight loss plan, I actually gained 2 pounds this week. I still can't fight the urge to eat in the evenings.

FACILITATOR 2: When was the most recent occurrence when you binged?

ELLEN: Last night.

FACILITATOR 2: OK, last night. Ellen, take a moment to imagine last night. Describe the scene to us.

ELLEN: *(sniffing)* It was a little after 8:00, and I was sitting in the living room watching a sappy movie on Lifetime TV. I know I shouldn't watch those, they're always about relationships and families, and they remind me what I don't have anymore.…

FACILITATOR 2: *(prompts Ellen to keep going)*

ELLEN: Well, the movie was actually about a family that was having problems because the oldest son was arrested and having trouble with the law. But that wasn't what made me sad. It was a scene where the mother and father had a moment of being really close, where they said that they would stick by each other no matter what and get through it.… *(trailing off)*

FACILITATOR 2: Ellen, what was running through your mind in that situation?

ELLEN: *(crying again)* That I'm all alone, that no one will ever be supportive of me like that.

MICHAEL: How did that make you want to eat, Ellen?

ELLEN: Well, at that point I was crying pretty hard. I wanted something to calm me down, but the empty apartment was just more depressing.

FACILITATOR 1: So you couldn't figure out a way to comfort yourself?

ELLEN: No, I couldn't. So I went to the fridge and defrosted a frozen cheesecake.

FACILITATOR 1: What was running through your mind as you were defrosting the cheesecake?

ELLEN: That it doesn't matter if I'm overweight, that I'm always going to be alone, so I might as well get what little pleasure out of life I can.

FACILITATOR 1: (turning to the group) Does anyone hear anything in the way she is thinking that Ellen might be able to address?

ALLISON: Well, she believes she's always going to be alone. Isn't that all-or-nothing thinking?

FACILITATOR 2: That certainly applies. When you hear the word always or never, that's a clue that all-or-nothing thinking might be at work.

BRIAN: That's strange because I thought it was a different cognitive distortion. I thought Ellen was catastrophizing because she doesn't know for sure that the future will be that bleak.

FACILITATOR 2: Excellent point, Brian. One thing to keep in mind as we identify and evaluate these thoughts is that more than one process can be at work. They aren't always mutually exclusive. Does anyone see any other unhelpful thinking going on here?

MICHAEL: I think "I might as well get a little pleasure out of life" is an example of a facilitating thought.

FACILITATOR 2: You got it. Ellen, here's an important question. Does eating a cheesecake when you're feeling lonely lead to getting a little pleasure out of life?

ELLEN: Well, yes, it calms me down, and I really love cheesecake.

MICHAEL: Yeah, Ellen, but how long does that last?

ELLEN: (tearful again) Not long. It just starts everything all over again. I'm guilty for ruining my diet. And I put myself down for being weak and alone.

FACILITATOR 1: This is an important lesson for all of us. You know that addictions are very, very powerful. I wouldn't be surprised if all of you have had facilitating thoughts like Ellen's—that you deserve a little bit of pleasure out of life. In theory, I don't disagree. You do deserve pleasure out of life. However, when you have that thought about your *addictions*, it is crucial for you to think about whether giving into the slip leads to pleasure. In most cases, as with Ellen, the pleasure is short-lived, and the consequences are guilt, shame, and being one step closer to a relapse.

In our experience, we have found that it is vitally important for facilitators to be familiar with common questions to facilitate the evaluation of situational cognitions, as displayed in Figure 7.3, and the circumstances under which particular questions are most relevant. They can then, in turn, model the use of these questions with their group members. For example, many patients express future-oriented thoughts that are usually associated with anxiety, such as Dave's thought that his girlfriend is going be pregnant, and if so, that she will be unable to contribute to running the household. Decatastrophizing questions are especially useful to pose in these situations, such as "Are you 100% sure of these consequences?"; "What is the likelihood that _____ will occur?"; "What's the best outcome? What's the worst outcome? What's the most realistic outcome?"; and "If _____ occurs, how bad will that be?" (J. S. Beck, 2011). When the future-oriented thoughts involve a prediction that they will not be able to withstand the urge to engage in addictive behavior, facilitators can help group members to brainstorm coping strategies for dealing with urges (see Chapter 8) and then estimate the likelihood of a slip when these skills are in place. Sometimes patients overgeneralize a slip as signifying a full-blown relapse (cf. L. C. Sobell & Sobell, 2011). In these cases, facilitators might ask them to evaluate the evidence that supports and refutes the statement (e.g., "I did have one slip, but I also have been coming to group for 3 months and have been able to stay abstinent during that time"), or to ask if one slip equals a relapse. It is important for the facilitator to pair these cognitive strategies with the coping skills discussed in Chapter 8 in order to help patients develop the tools to manage urges and cravings. While engaging in this process, facilitators take every opportunity to consolidate group members' learning by encouraging them to ask these questions of themselves.

Although there is often a "grain of truth" in situational cognitions, in most cases group members have exaggerated them in some way, which in turn leads to elevated levels of distress. However, there are some circumstances in which group members' situational cognitions largely reflect reality, particularly when these cognitions are descriptive. In Allison's case, it is very likely that she *will* indeed come home to a house full of smoke after work because her husband and mother-in-law have made it clear to her that they will not refrain from smoking in the house. If the facilitators were to encourage her fellow group members to question the validity of her appraisal of this situation, she would likely feel misunderstood and judged. In such a case, the facilitators might validate the difficulty of this situation and gently prompt the group member to consider whether it is *helpful* or *useful* to be focusing on such thoughts and images. That is, facilitators create an environment for the group member to question the utility of his or her cognition and identify cognitions that are more helpful in promoting active coping and problem solving. Consider the following vignette:

ALLISON: I hate going home from work.

ELLEN: I can imagine how much you hate going home from work, Allison. You're putting so much work into quitting smoking, and it seems like your husband and mother-in-law are doing everything they can to set you up for failure.

ALLISON: (*giving Ellen a look of gratitude*) Yeah, that's it exactly.

FACILITATOR 1: Allison, imagine that it is the end of the day and you are about to go home. What runs through your mind?

ALLISON: I see my kitchen table, with my husband and mother-in-law sitting at it doing nothing but smoking. The ashtray is filled with cigarette butts.

FACILITATOR 1: When this image is conjured up in your mind, what emotion do you experience?

ALLISON: A lot of dread. Some anxiety, too, because I know that all of the smoking cues will be right in my face as soon as I walk in the door, and I don't know if I can resist.

MICHAEL: (*shaking his head in sympathy*)

FACILITATOR 1: This seems like a difficult situation to be in, as you are making positive gains to stop smoking once and for all. How often do you experience this image right before going home from work?

ALLISON: Every day. And every day there is the dread.

FACILITATOR 2: How helpful is it for you to focus on this image?

ALLISON: I don't get what you mean.

FACILITATOR 2: Well, do you feel good when you have this image? Does it help you to prepare for your urges to smoke?

ALLISON: No, it does just the opposite. I feel deflated. I feel worn down, like I'm tired of fighting them all the time.

FACILITATOR 2: It sounds like the situation is not likely to change anytime soon. But one thing you can change is the thought or image you focus on at the end of the day. Can you think of anything that would help you to feel less deflated, less worn down, and instead more powerful in resisting urges to smoke?

ALLISON: Hmmm, I haven't thought about that before. Maybe I can picture myself at the doctor's office, getting a clean bill of health?

FACILITATOR 1: What does everyone think of this strategy?

ELLEN: I think that's a good idea. Really focusing on the good coming out of your choice to stop smoking, rather than on your husband and mother-in-law. Maybe I'll try this, too. Like, I can imagine myself being able to walk up the stairs without huffing and puffing.

MICHAEL: And maybe both of you can think about all the things that you can do with your life if you kick your bad habits.

(Allison and Ellen speak simultaneously about Michael's suggestion being a good one.)

The vignettes presented thus far are instances in which facilitators and group members ask questions to help group members gain perspective on the accuracy and helpfulness of their situational cognitions. In order to ensure that group members can use these strategies in their daily lives, it is crucial that facilitators work collaboratively with group members to develop creative ways to internalize this process of questioning. In the following vignette, the facilitators attempt to consolidate learning about the questioning process:

FACILITATOR 1: You've all had another day of hard work. Can each of you tell me, in your own words, what we've done today and how you are going to use this in your life outside of session?

ALLISON: I learned that I have to find ways to recognize when my thinking is getting me in trouble and really ask myself if it is worth it.

FACILITATOR 1: And what if you decide that it is not worth it? That it will just make you feel worse or make you vulnerable to a slip or a lapse?

ALLISON: Then I have to do something different. This level of dread cannot go on forever; it's making me miserable.

BRIAN: I agree with Allison. And I also think I really need to think through the short- and long-term consequences of going to the casino. Like the fact that there is only a very small possibility that

I will win big, and that I'll dig a hole that is even deeper if I blow all of my money.

DAVE: *(sighing)* I guess I need to have my girlfriend take a pregnancy test before I drive myself crazy.

BRIAN: *(patting Dave on the back as a sign of support)*

FACILITATOR 2: Excellent conclusions. We considered lots of different ways to question our thoughts in group today. Which questions stick out as the most useful in evaluating unhelpful thoughts?

ELLEN: You just said the word unhelpful. I really need to ask myself if it is helping me to dwell on certain things in my life.

BRIAN: For me, it's what are the consequences?

MICHAEL: In my time in the group, I've found that I use the evidence question the most. Like what is the evidence that life will be less satisfying without sex outside of my marriage? 'Cause I've found the opposite, that life is *better* without all of the sneaking around and guilt.

Responding to Situational Cognitions

Throughout the course of their participation in CTAGs, group members learn that there is a strong association between negative automatic thoughts and images and distressing emotions. They also learn that there is a strong association between outcome expectancies and facilitating thoughts and the likelihood of giving in to urges or cravings. In order to increase the likelihood that group members engage in healthy, adaptive behaviors rather than unhealthy, maladaptive behaviors, it is important that they respond actively to their situational cognitions.

After group members elicit inaccurate and unhelpful situational cognitions, facilitators guide them in using the process of questioning described in the previous section to develop an *alternative response*. Alternative responses are more balanced thoughts and images that are constructed after group members identify and evaluate situational cognitions. Other names for alternative responses are *adaptive responses* and *balanced responses*. Often, they can be constructed simply by answering the question posed in evaluating the situational cognition. For example, if a group member has the thought, "I won't be able to resist a drink at the office holiday party," one of the facilitators or another group member might ask about the likelihood of that event occurring or to list the evidence that supports and refutes that statement. The group member might respond, "It's not very likely that I will let myself have a drink, as I've already been to two office parties where I did not drink." The alternative response is not meant to be uniformly positive or optimistic—in fact, such a response has the potential to be just as unrealistic as the situational cognition that is the focus of the exercise. Instead, the alternative response is constructed on the basis of all of the available pieces of evidence, acknowledging that the situation might be difficult or less than perfect, but also accounting for the group member's abilities to handle adversity, the possibility to find wisdom, or the balance between the situation's positive and negative aspects. The following vignette illustrates the process of constructing alternative responses in Ellen's situation. Recall that the group had just identified the fact that getting pleasure from addictive behaviors is short-lived and often leads to guilt and shame:

FACILITATOR 1: Ellen, let's imagine that you are in a similar situation tonight. You're home alone watching a television movie, and something in the movie triggers feelings of loneliness. On a scale of 0–100, how much sadness would you be experiencing, with 100 being the most sadness you've ever experienced?

ELLEN: Oh, a lot. I'd say a 90 or 95. It's been really bad lately.

FACILITATOR 1: And after struggling with this distress for awhile, you say to yourself "I might as well get some pleasure out of life" and contemplate heading to the freezer to defrost a cheesecake. How might you handle that facilitating thought?

ELLEN: I could ask myself the likelihood that I actually *would* get pleasure out of eating cheesecake?

FACILITATOR 1: Now using that question, how might you construct an alternative response?

ELLEN: (*tentatively*) I could say that there isn't much likelihood at all that I would get pleasure out of it?

FACILITATOR 1: You could say that. On that same 0–100 scale, how much sadness would you be experiencing after acknowledging that alternative response?

ELLEN: (*shaking her head*) I still think it would be just as high. I'd still be sad.

FACILITATOR 1: (*to the group*) This illustrates the importance of coming up with a *compelling* alternative response. It is very true that Ellen probably won't get much long-term pleasure out of eating the cheesecake. But it seems that this alternative response is not as powerful as the addiction-related thought. What else could Ellen add to the alternative response to make it work in reducing the likelihood that she would get up and make the cheesecake?

MICHAEL: Maybe she could look at the consequences and then say something like, "Even though eating the cheesecake might give me pleasure in the short term, I will feel guilty about eating it in the long run. And by not eating the cheesecake, I have taken an important step in my recovery?"

FACILITATOR 1: Ellen, if you were to say that to yourself, how much sadness would you experience on the 0–100 scale?

ELLEN: Actually, I think that might work, it might go down to like a 40. The sadness would still be there regardless of whether I do or do not eat the cheesecake because I still have a lot of personal issues to deal with. But at least I can consider myself a little bit stronger because I resisted the binge.

Notice that Facilitator 1 encouraged Ellen to assign a number indicating the intensity of her emotion, both when she identified her situational cognition as well as after she constructed an alternative response. Rating the intensity of emotions serves several purposes. First, it provides information to facilitators about the severity of the group member's distress, which serves as a guide in determining the amount of time to spend addressing a particular issue. Second, it helps group members to differentiate among their experiences. Some group members have difficulty tolerating distress and appraise every situation as "awful" or "the worst." Assigning varying levels of intensity to their emotional reactions provides evidence that, though distressing, not all situations are intolerable and, thereby, necessitate engagement in the addictive behavior. Finally, the ratings provide evidence for the usefulness of constructing alternative responses. When group members observe that the intensity of their distress decreases after constructing an alternative response, they come to realize that the exercise is helpful, and their motivation to use such cognitive strategies in the future is increased.

The Thought Record, described earlier in this chapter, can be expanded to include practice in generating alternative responses and noticing associated outcomes. The *Six-Column Thought Record* (see Form 7.2 at the end of the chapter) includes the same four columns as the Four-Column Thought Record—situations or triggers, situational cognitions, emotions, and behaviors—as well as two new columns: alternative response and outcome. The alternative response column allows group members to record a new self-statement that reflects the conclusion drawn from the questioning process. The outcome column allows group members to record what is different as a result of constructing an alternative response. In most instances, it is expected that a compelling alternative response will (1) decrease the intensity of negative emotional experiences, as it did with Ellen; (2) increase the likelihood of more positive emotional experiences, such as pride; and (3) increase the likelihood of adaptive behavior, such as not engaging in addictive behavior, not remaining in the presence of "people, places, and things" that serve as a trigger, and implementing an adaptive coping skill. The Six-Column Thought Record can be completed by group members in session, and/or it can serve as a homework assignment.

Sometimes it becomes evident that particular situational cognitions occur repeatedly in particular group members. In these instances, it is helpful for facilitators to encourage the use of *coping cards*. A coping card is a 3″×5″ index card with helpful strategies that group members can consult in times of distress in order to respond to inaccurate and unhelpful situational cognitions. For example, facilitators might assist group members in identifying typical outcome expectancies related to urges and cravings, jotting those cognitions on their coping cards, and constructing alternative responses that are also recorded on the coping card (see Figure 7.4). Group members can carry coping cards with them in their wallets, purses, or planners (or even in their cigarette boxes if they are still smoking) and can consult them when they have difficulty responding to the typical situational cognitions that occur in their daily lives. Coping cards can also be created and accessed electronically, such as in the 'notes' app on a smartphone.

WORKING WITH BELIEFS

As described in Chapters 2 and 5, basic beliefs are the most central, fundamental ideas that people have about themselves, the world, and/or the future. In most instances, the nature of the automatic thought elicited in a particular situation is determined, in part, by an individual's basic belief.

Automatic Thought: I'm never going to kick this habit. It's too hard.

Alternative Response: It's true that it is hard to kick addictions. But there is a lot of evidence that I've been successful already. I attend the CTAG on a weekly basis. I've only slipped twice in the past 6 months. And it would be more helpful to focus on all of the positive consequences of kicking the habit—improved health, improved financial situation, and improved relationships.

FIGURE 7.4. Sample coping card.

Addiction-related beliefs are fundamental ideas about engagement in addictive behavior, and in a similar manner as basic beliefs, fuel the nature of the specific outcome expectancy that is activated in the face of a trigger. Group members can develop skills to successfully evaluate situational cognitions, but if maladaptive or unhelpful basic beliefs and addiction-related beliefs are not also modified, then they are at risk of continuing to make faulty appraisals of events in their environment and being prone to having slips and lapses when they encounter a trigger. That is, the modification of unhelpful beliefs is necessary for long-term emotional well-being. In this section, we examine ways to identify basic beliefs and addiction-related beliefs, as well as strategies for modifying beliefs that are unhelpful.

Identifying Beliefs

Facilitators will have begun to develop hypotheses about group members' beliefs as they develop cognitive case conceptualizations (see Chapter 5). However, it is important for group members to identify their basic beliefs and addiction-related beliefs on their own through guided questioning, rather than being told by facilitators what their beliefs are. Realization of beliefs is a powerful therapeutic moment for most group members, and it often signals a "turning point" in treatment because it provides a coherent framework for understanding their struggles and a clear pathway for change.

It takes more probing to identify a belief than it does to identify a situational cognition, as it is assumed that situational cognitions are at the surface of awareness, whereas beliefs are ingrained and not always easy to articulate. One way to identify a group member's beliefs is to discern one or more themes associated with the situational cognitions that he or she reports. Another way is to ask group members directly about the messages that they received as a child and the degree to which those messages influence them as adults. This approach is illustrated by the dialogue with Michael in Chapter 5, in which the facilitators learned that Michael developed the idea that he is incompetent and not "manly" because he did not share the same interests as his father and his brother. A third way to identify beliefs is to lead the group member through a verbal exercise designed to probe beyond the content of the situational cognition into the meaning behind it. This approach is called the *downward arrow technique* (A. T. Beck et al., 1979; Burns, 1980). There are often several layers of meaning associated with a group member's cognition, and the facilitators might need to ask the question "And what did *that* mean to you?" several times before arriving upon the belief. The following vignette focuses on the meaning of Dave's automatic thought about not having any fun in the event that his girlfriend is pregnant and has a baby:

DAVE: I was just like, "Screw it. I might as well go get drunk because I'm not going to have any fun in about 7 months."

FACILITATOR 2: Dave, you seem visibly agitated right now. Obviously, the idea about not having fun anymore is a powerful one to you. What does it mean to you that you're not going to have any fun?

DAVE: What do you mean by that, what does it mean not to have fun anymore? It means life will be boring!

FACILITATOR 2: It means life will be boring. (*pausing*) One thing that jumps to mind for me is that a lot of people's lives might not be that exciting, particularly as they get older and have more responsibility, but they seem to get a great deal of satisfaction and comfort from that. In fact, we've heard Michael say this very thing as he reflects on his life after giving up his sex addiction. Help me understand how your situation is different.

DAVE: (*exasperated*) I'm just, I'm just … not ready for this.

FACILITATOR 2: And what does that mean about you, or about your life?

DAVE: I'm not sure I want to be in this relationship, in this situation. I was just starting to figure things out, finally been sober enough to have my head on straight, and now this.

FACILITATOR 2: So you were finally getting your life together, finally starting to think about what *you* want in the long term, and now there is the possibility that you will be faced with a responsibility that you aren't sure you would have chosen.

DAVE: (*softly*) Yeah, exactly.

FACILITATOR 2: And what does this *mean* to you?

DAVE: (*hesitating, head in hands*) It means I'm trapped. Forever. I've been trapped my whole life, trapped in a stupid trailer park because my parents couldn't get it together to hold down steady work, trapped in this stupid town because I never finished high school and wasn't able to get out, and now, trapped in a relationship with someone I know I don't want to be with for the rest of my life.

FACILITATOR 2: (*gently*) So would you say this belief of being trapped is a belief that pervades much of the way you approach things in your life?

DAVE: (*looking surprised*) Yeah, I would say so.

FACILITATOR 2: I think we just hit upon one of your basic beliefs.

(*Facilitators initiate a discussion with group members to consider the value of probing about the meaning in order to identify their own unique basic beliefs.)*

Modifying Beliefs

Many of the same strategies used to modify situational cognitions can also be used to modify maladaptive and unhelpful beliefs. For example, facilitators can guide group members in identifying evidence that supports and refutes a belief or in examining the advantages and disadvantages of holding a particular belief in order to draw a conclusion about the degree to which it is helpful or functional. However, it is important to realize that beliefs are rarely modified fully after one attempt to evaluate their validity and usefulness because they are deeply rooted, are associated with intense emotions, and have been in existence for much of an individual's life. The following are three specific strategies that can be used to modify maladaptive and unhelpful beliefs:

Cognitive Continuum

The cognitive continuum is a strategy for modifying unhelpful beliefs that are rigid, absolute, and extreme (e.g., "I'm a failure," "I'm worthless"; J. S. Beck, 2011). Facilitators guide group members in creating a continuum ranging from favorable to unfavorable manifestations of the belief, identifying examples of people who reflect various anchors along the continuum, and realistically placing themselves at an accurate point along the continuum. When group members objectively examine where they stand along the continuum, they usually find that they fall in the middle or even a favorable range along the continuum, rather than at the unfavorable end of the continuum. This strategy was particularly useful for Michael, who continues to struggle with the basic belief that he is an incompetent man:

> FACILITATOR 1: Michael, I'd like to do an exercise with you to help you evaluate realistically whether you are truly incompetent. Are you game?
>
> MICHAEL: *(nodding)*
>
> FACILITATOR 1: Are the rest of you willing to jump in and help me?
>
> ELLEN: Definitely, because I have never thought that Michael is incompetent. I think you have a lot more going for you than many of us.
>
> *(Other group members nod their heads.)*
>
> FACILITATOR 1: What I'd like to do is examine in greater detail this

concept of competence. First of all, Michael, can you tell me what you mean by incompetent? Incompetent in what sense?

MICHAEL: I know it sounds stupid, but incompetent in terms of being a man.

FACILITATOR 1: And how do you define being "a man"?

MICHAEL: Well, I guess most traditional things. Having a good job, making enough money to be comfortable, taking care of your family.

FACILITATOR 1: (*sensing there is more to it in Michael's situation*) Those are important pieces. I wonder if there are also some other pieces, on the basis of the messages you got from your father when you were younger? Has anyone else heard Michael refer to other things that could go into being a man?

BRIAN: You seem to feel guilty about not being very handy around the house, like fixing the car or doing repairs around the house.

MICHAEL: Yeah, I think you're right. And being a man also meant controlling your emotions—never showing weakness.

FACILITATOR 1: OK, we've identified five components that you believe go into being a competent man—job, money, taking care of family, being handy, and controlling your emotions. What I'd like you to do is to think of the person who most represents this concept of being a competent man.

MICHAEL: Hmmm ... well ... I guess my cousin Heath. He grew up in the same kind of household—his dad is my father's brother. He's really successful. He owns a lot of garages, so he has a lot of money. And he actually built his own house. My family looks at him like he's a king.

FACILITATOR 1: OK, so we have your cousin at one end of the continuum. (*drawing a line on the whiteboard, with 0% anchoring the left end point, and 100% with the name "Heath" anchoring the right end point*) Who might be at the other end of the spectrum, someone who you don't view as a competent man at all?

MICHAEL: (*laughing*) I guess that would be another cousin of mine, Paul. He's really out there, really artsy, has dreadlocks, and wears bright-colored robes and all. (*chuckling.*) Woo-boy, you should see how my family reacts when he goes to our family events!

(*Group also chuckles.*)

FACILITATOR 1: (*writing down "Paul" anchoring the left end point*) What do the rest of you think? Are these accurate anchors at each end of the continuum of competence?

ALLISON: I know you're focusing just on people you know, Michael. But what about a homeless man, or a man who's in jail for murdering somebody? Men like that don't have jobs or money. And they're not taking care of their family.

MICHAEL: I never thought of that. I guess they'd have to be even worse than Paul. Maybe in the negative range!

(*Group laughs.*)

FACILITATOR 2: It looks like we have to rearrange our continuum. Shall we put homeless men and jailed murders at 0%?

MICHAEL: (*nodding*)

FACILITATOR 2: And where, then would Paul go?

MICHAEL: I guess there probably are a lot of guys who are even less competent than Paul. Guys who are unemployed, don't pay child support, you name it. So maybe Paul is more like at 25%.

FACILITATOR 1: (*making a 25% anchor along the continuum and writing "Paul" and then erasing "Paul" from 0% and writing "homeless man/jailed murderer"*)

DAVE: (*a bit sarcastically*) Is your cousin Heath *really* the most competent man in the world? What about the president of the United States?

MICHAEL: Well, I don't know if the president knows how to fix cars or not, but I guess all that he has accomplished makes that part of being a man irrelevant. He's a competent man any way you look at it.

FACILITATOR 2: So should we put the president at 100%?

MICHAEL: (*nodding*)

BRIAN: (*joking*) I'm not sure that everyone would agree that the president should be listed as 100% competent!

(*Group erupts in laughter.*)

FACILITATOR 2: (*smiling*) Well, if we say the president or someone as accomplished as the president is at 100%, where, then, would Heath fall?

MICHAEL: I don't know, let's say, 90%.

FACILITATOR 1: (*making the appropriate adjustments along the continuum*) At what point along this continuum, using percentages, does "incompetent" start?

MICHAEL: I don't know, maybe 50%?

FACILITATOR 1: OK, we'll write that up here for now. (*putting a tick mark in the center of the line, writing "50%," and writing*)

"*Incompetent*") For the sake of argument, let's identify someone who is right in the middle of Heath and Paul. Can you think of who that might be?

MICHAEL: Umm, maybe my coworker, Jamie. He obviously has a steady job at my law firm. And he's able to make enough money to support his family, and they have a house and all. But I do know that he has some debt, which makes things tight for his family.

FACILITATOR 1: And does he do any work with his hands, you know, like repairs around the house?

MICHAEL: Not that I know of.

FACILITATOR 1: (*writing "Jamie" under "50%"*) You said a minute ago that "incompetent" starts at 50%. Do you view Jamie as incompetent?

MICHAEL: Oh no, I wouldn't say "incompetent." Just maybe that he could be handling things a little better.

FACILITATOR 2: So then, where does "incompetent" start?

MICHAEL: I see your point. I guess it's not true that like 50% of all men would be considered incompetent. So let me say that "incompetent" starts at 25%.

FACILITATOR 1: (*placing a tick mark at approximately 25% along the continuum, writing "Incompetent," and erasing "Incompetent" from the 50% mark*) Michael, where do you fall on the continuum, relative to Heath, Jamie, and Paul?

MICHAEL: (*shaking his head in disbelief*) You know, before doing this I would have put myself at like 20%, hell, maybe even 0%. But looking at this, I would actually put myself a little above Jamie, maybe at like 55 or 60%. I have a more senior position than him, and I don't have as much debt. I think I do more for my family. And even Paul is a little bit competent, so maybe I have to move the cutoff for incompetence down even further.

ELLEN: See, Michael? I told you that we all think you're very competent, although, personally, I think you should put yourself higher than 55 or 60%.

ALLISON: Yeah, me too.

BRIAN: Me too, definitely.

FACILITATOR 2: So how accurate is it to call someone who falls at the 55 or 60% mark incompetent?

MICHAEL: I guess it isn't. I guess there are some things I have going for me that show I'm a competent man even if I don't know the first thing about working with my hands.

FACILITATOR 1: I appreciate that everyone chipped in and helped out with this. Michael seems to have gained a lot of insight about the degree to which his basic belief that he is incompetent is accurate. What have the rest of you taken away from this exercise?

BRIAN: You guys know that I have been feeling like a complete loser lately. So I probably also would have put myself at 0%. But I guess my life is going better than the homeless man and jailed murderer.

ALLISON: Yeah, it's real easy to get sucked into "poor me"; I have it worse than anyone. But if you really take the time to look at where you stand as compared to everyone in this world—not just the people who seem like they're doing better than you—then you realize that you do have some things going for you.

FACILITATOR 2: And how might that help you with your addiction?

ALLISON: For me, it shows me that I am stronger than a lot of people and that I can use that strength to kick the habit once and for all.

This vignette illustrates many important techniques to ensure the successful application of the cognitive continuum. First, Facilitator 1 spent some time helping Michael to define the specific components of being a competent man. This step is important because many group members have vague, global beliefs that are not well articulated but that they take as fact. When they begin to see that there are many components to being competent, successful, or worthwhile, they realize that they are ignoring the components on which they are doing quite well. Second, the facilitators invited Michael and the other group members to identify realistic anchors at various points along the continuum. As was illustrated in this vignette, it is helpful to complete this exercise using media that is readily erasable, as the anchors that are originally identified are often shifted once group members carefully evaluate them. Third, Facilitator 1 helped Michael to think realistically about the point along the continuum where incompetence starts. Finally, both facilitators invited group members to reflect on the manner in which the exercise applied to their basic beliefs as well as to their addictive behavior.

Behavioral Experiments

From our experience, verbal and written strategies to modify beliefs and situational cognitions that reflect those beliefs are a tremendous resource for group members who are vulnerable to urges, cravings, and unpleasant moods such as depression and anxiety. Over time and with practice,

patients learn to "catch" their cognitive distortions and think systematically before making an exaggerated appraisal of difficult situations. In a
sense, they become their own cognitive therapists. Another strategy for
responding to problematic cognitions goes beyond the verbal or written
exercise of asking questions and constructing alternative responses or new
beliefs. *Behavioral experiments* are strategies in which patients actively test
out their negative cognitions in their own environments. Nothing is more
powerful than observing firsthand that your appraisal of yourself or of a
situation is too simplistic, incorrect, or exaggerated.

Beliefs are typically pervasive and abstract; thus, it is difficult, if not
impossible, to devise a behavioral experiment to test the validity of a belief
in its entirety. Nevertheless, behavioral experiments are effective tools in
addressing beliefs when the belief is broken down into manageable, concrete
components. For example, Ellen has the basic belief that she is unlovable,
such that she believes that she is bound to be rejected and to be alone for
the rest of her life. One area of her life where these beliefs manifest themselves is in her relationship with her daughter. Because her daughter lives in
another area of the country, they rarely have telephone conversations, and
when they do communicate, Ellen views their interactions as unfulfilling.
When she thinks about her daughter, she has automatic thoughts such as
"She will be unresponsive," or "She's never going to let me into her life." To
begin to test the idea that she would never have a meaningful relationship
with her daughter, the facilitators encouraged Ellen to call her daughter on
the telephone and use some of the relationship-building skills discussed in
Chapter 8 to evaluate the validity of the prediction that her daughter would
be unresponsive. Over time, a number of these experiments were devised to
test out her predictions and beliefs about her relationship with her daughter, and subsequently, her relationships with other individuals who had the
potential to be close others in her life. Ellen accumulated more and more
evidence to refute the idea that she is bound to be rejected and alone for the
rest of her life, and thereby unlovable.

It is important for behavioral experiments to be designed in a manner
that creates a "win–win" situation for group members. Many behavioral
experiments, like Ellen's, involve other people, and facilitators, of course,
cannot predict how others will behave. When Ellen implemented the early
behavioral experiments to make contact with her daughter, the facilitators
were not sure that her daughter would, indeed, be responsive. Thus, the
group helped to prepare Ellen for both positive and negative outcomes. A
positive outcome, such as her daughter showing interest in conversation,
was construed as evidence to refute the prediction that her daughter would
be unresponsive and to soften the belief that she is unlovable. However, a
negative outcome, such as her daughter showing little interest in the conversation, had the potential to make Ellen even more depressed and could,

potentially, serve as a trigger for binge eating. Thus, the group worked with Ellen to develop coping skills to implement in the event that her daughter showed little interest in the conversation, which could then refute beliefs associated with Ellen's low self-efficacy (e.g., "I have no control over my eating when I am upset").

It is tempting for facilitators to devise behavioral experiments that involve exposing group members to triggers to engage in addictive behaviors in order to give them evidence that they can successfully implement the strategies that they are learning in treatment to avoid a slip or a lapse. However, we would advise against this experiment, as it is very risky (cf. Monti et al., 2002). Virtually all intervention approaches for people with addictive disorders uniformly recommend that they stay away from "people, places, and things" that trigger engagement in addictive behavior, so it would be unwise to put group members at unnecessary risk. However, group members will undoubtedly come across "people, places, and things" on various occasions in their daily lives. If they successfully manage urges and cravings, then facilitators can draw similar conclusions as ones that are often concluded after structured behavioral experiments—that group members can indeed cope and make sound decisions in their lives.

Development of Control Beliefs

Control beliefs are beliefs that decrease the likelihood that an individual will engage in addictive behavior by focusing on his or her ability to withstand the urge and implement an adaptive response. In other words, it is a belief that counteracts an addiction-related belief. Some control beliefs reflect a strong sense of self-efficacy (e.g., "I am a strong person who can overcome addiction"). Other control beliefs reflect the advantages of overcoming addiction (e.g., "Life is more fulfilling without (*insert name of addiction*)") or the disadvantages or consequences of engaging in addictive behavior (e.g., "(*Insert name of addiction*) makes like less fulfilling, not more fulfilling"). Typical questions facilitators can ask to guide the development of control beliefs include "What are the advantages of being free of your addiction?," "What are the disadvantages or consequences of your addiction,?" "Now that you have developed strategies for coping, what kind of a person are you?," and "What else could you do to achieve the same end as the addictive behavior?" (A. T. Beck et al., 1993).

An important point to remember about control beliefs is that they need to be practiced over and over. Anticipatory outcome expectancies, relief-oriented outcome expectancies, and facilitating thoughts are especially powerful and easily activated in situations that involve triggers for addictive behaviors because they have been overpracticed. They undoubtedly will override control beliefs unless the latter are firmly solidified. Thus, it is incumbent on facilitators to be creative in reinforcing these new beliefs. Similar to the strategy described previously for responding to automatic thoughts, facilitators can encourage patients to record their control beliefs on a coping card to consult during times of temptation. In addition, they can write a list of the disadvantages for engaging in the addictive behavior on the card. Facilitators also can spend time in *imagery rehearsal* with group members. In such an exercise, facilitators can lead members through an imagery exercise designed to activate cravings and urges. Subsequently, they can encourage group members to rehearse their control beliefs, either mentally or out loud. Facilitators can obtain an estimate of the degree of craving before and after activating the control beliefs on a 0–100 scale in the same manner as emotions are rated before and after the construction of an alternative response.

SUMMARY

Unhelpful basic beliefs often set the context for automatic thoughts and images to be activated in specific situations, which in turn lead to emotional distress and maladaptive behavioral responses. Unhelpful addictions-related beliefs often set the context for anticipatory and relief-oriented outcome expectancies and facilitating thoughts to be activated in response to a trigger. Individuals who participate in CTAGs can develop skills to identify and evaluate these situational cognitions as well as to identify and modify the beliefs that drive the activation of these cognitions (see Figure 7.5 for a summary of these strategies). When group members describe problematic situations, facilitators might ask them what was running through their mind at that time and follow with a question designed for group members to distance themselves from their situational cognition and evaluate the situation in an adaptive, balanced manner. Group members can respond to situational cognitions by constructing alternative responses, which, in some instances, are recorded on a Thought Record or a coping card. Facilitators can guide group members in identifying their underlying beliefs by prompting them to assess the meaning of a particular situation. These beliefs can be modified by examining the evidence for and against them over time, completing a cognitive continuum, completing behavioral experiments, and/or developing control beliefs.

It is important to acknowledge that this chapter contains only a handful of the basic cognitive therapy strategies that have been developed to identify, evaluate, and modify thoughts and beliefs. Readers who gain expertise in applying these strategies will have the tools to conduct a successful

---

SITUATIONAL COGNITIONS

- Step 1: *Identify situational cognition.*

    Group discussion

    Four-Column Thought Record

- Step 2: *Evaluate situational cognition using focused questioning.*

- Step 3: *Respond to situational cognition by constructing an alternative response.*

    Group discussion

    Six-Column Thought Record

    Coping card

BELIEFS

- Step 1: *Identify belief.*

    Group discussion

    Themes reflected in situational cognitions

    Messages received as a child

    Downward arrow technique

- Step 2: *Modify belief.*

    Examine evidence that supports old and new belief over time

    Cognitive continuum

    Behavioral experiment

    Development of control beliefs

FIGURE 7.5. Summary of strategies to modify situational cognitions and beliefs.

CTAG. However, group facilitators also can have the leeway to adapt other cognitive therapy strategies that they encounter in reading, supervision, and continuing education to a group format for patients with addictions. We encourage readers to keep abreast of current literature on cognitive therapy as well as to have standard resources such as J. S. Beck's (2011) *Cognitive Behavior Therapy: Basics and Beyond*, A. T. Beck et al.'s (1993) *Cognitive Therapy of Substance Abuse*, and J. S. Beck's (2005) *Cognitive Therapy for Challenging Problems: What to Do When the Basics Don't Work*.

FORM 7.1. Four-Column Thought Record

Situation or Trigger What happened? What prompted the urges and cravings?	Thought/Outcome Expectancy What thought(s) ran through your mind? What did that situation or trigger mean to you?	Emotion What feeling(s) did you experience? (Rate on a scale of 0–100)	Behavior What did you do as a result of the thought and emotion?

FORM 7.2. Six-Column Thought Record

Situation or Trigger	Thought/Outcome Expectancy	Emotion	Behavior	Alternative Response	Outcome
What happened? What prompted the urges and cravings?	What thought(s) ran through your mind? What did that situation or trigger mean to you?	What feeling(s) did you experience? (Rate on a scale of 0–100)	What did you do as a result of the thought and emotion?	What balanced conclusion do you draw after questioning the unhelpful thought?	How much do you believe the original thought now? How intense are the feelings now? What will you do differently now?

CHAPTER 8 | Developing Coping Skills

Many experts believe that addictive behavior is a maladaptive way to manage stress (e.g., Monti et al., 2002). It is often the case that people who struggle with addictions lack the skills to manage stress, have a vulnerability to experience the effects of stress especially acutely, and/or are dealing with an inordinate number of stressors in their lives. It follows, then, that they could benefit from the acquisition and practice of skills to cope with stress. According to Monti et al., stress results "from an imbalance between environmental demands and an individual's resources," and "coping is an attempt to meet the demand in a way that restores balance and equilibrium" (p. 3).

A focus on the development of coping skills provides cognitive and behavioral strategies that complement the strategies described in Chapter 7 to manage cravings, urges, emotional distress, and other consequences of addictions. They are meant to be used *in conjunction* with the tools to evaluate thoughts and beliefs. For example, a group member might replace a maladaptive thought such as "I deserve to get high" with an alternative response such as "I deserve to live a happy, healthy life, and to do that I need to stay sober." The coping skills described in this chapter will help group members to comply with that adaptive alternative response and will provide evidence to support the notion that they can successfully manage cravings and facilitating thoughts.

The coping skill or skills that are targeted in any one session is decided upon by the facilitators after getting a sense of group members' concerns that are brought up in the introductions. Thus, it is important for facilitators to have a strong grasp on the wide array of coping skills described in this chapter and come prepared with the knowledge and materials to focus on particular coping skills as they are warranted. In the vignette of group introductions presented in Chapter 6, it quickly became evident to the facilitators that a number of group members were struggling with difficulties in their close relationships. To respond to these concerns, the facilitators verbally noted that a theme was emerging from the introductions and linked it to the concerns expressed by the remaining group members who had not yet given their introductions. In doing so, the facilitators were cognizant to weave a coherent thread across group members' difficulties and make explicit the manner in which the topic that would be targeted in the remainder of the session—repairing close relationships—was relevant to each of them.

In many instances, discussion of coping skills is a time that allows seasoned group members to share their triumphs and difficulties with new group members. When the group is focusing on a particular coping skill, those who have had experience in implementing the skill can share insights about ways in which it works well and ways in which it does not. These learning opportunities are effective in allowing seasoned group members to develop a sense of worth, in that they have valuable opinions to share with others (i.e., altruism). These instances also model to newer group members that the coping skills are effective, thereby enhancing new group members' sense of optimism regarding their own potential for progress (i.e., instillation of hope).

CTAG facilitators will invariably encounter instances in which one or more group members express skepticism about the coping skills, suggesting that they are not "buying in." For example, sometimes group members dismiss coping skills presented by the facilitators as being too simplistic or as not being powerful enough to counter urges and cravings. At other times, group members exhibit a sense of hopelessness, which interferes with their motivation to practice the coping skills being discussed. In these cases, facilitators can use the cognitive strategies described in Chapter 7, asking group members a question such as "When I make the suggestion to _____ when you experience an urge or a craving, what runs through your mind?" This strategy allows facilitators to identify negative thoughts about the coping skills and evaluate their validity. One way to overcome skepticism and/or hopelessness about the skill is to devise a behavioral experiment, such that group members monitor their mood, level of cravings, or whatever they are trying to modify before and after they implement the skill and use those ratings as evidence to evaluate the skill's effectiveness. Thus, the process of evaluating thoughts and beliefs is not only useful for modifying the manner in which group members view situations that they experience in their lives, but it is equally as useful for addressing obstacles that arise in practicing coping skills during sessions.

Figure 8.1 summarizes coping skills in six main areas that are often incorporated into CTAGs: (1) skills to manage urges and cravings; (2) skills to repair existing close relationships; (3) skills to develop new, healthy relationships; (4) skills to manage unpleasant emotions; (5) skills to improve problem solving; and (6) skills to lead a healthy lifestyle. Space does not allow us to discuss the full array of coping skills that is helpful to patients who struggle with addictions. CTAG facilitators need not be limited to the skills presented in this chapter and may integrate other skills from other cognitive behavioral interventions, clinical experience, and ongoing supervision.

MANAGING URGES AND CRAVINGS

The question that is posed most frequently by group members is, "How do I cope with my urges and cravings?" Group members who have been sober for months, and even years, continue to report that they experience urges and cravings on occasion. These experiences can be quite discouraging for group members and often lead to negative thoughts such as "I will never get over this" or "Life will always be like this." Thus, skills to manage urges and cravings are necessary to instill hope in group members that they will be able to successfully manage their addiction and live a quality life.

Distraction

Distraction is one straightforward strategy for managing urges and cravings. According to A. T. Beck et al. (1993), the goal of distraction is to shift patients' focus from their internal sensations, including thoughts, emotions, and physiological reactions, to something in their external environment. That is, distraction exercises help patients to move their focus from their craving onto something else that will hold their attention. In the language of the TTM (Prochaska & DiClemente, 2005), distraction can be regarded as stimulus control because it allows group members to manage important internal states that increase the likelihood of addictive behavior.

Distraction can take many forms. It can be primarily a cognitive or mental activity, such that patients focus their mind on pleasant images or an activity that requires cognitive resources, like reading, doing a puzzle, or simply describing all of their surroundings in detail in order to fully appreciate their external (vs. internal) environments. It can be an interpersonal activity such as calling a friend or sponsor. It can be a change of environment, such as going for a walk or drive or going to an environment that is not associated with the addiction, such as a museum. It can be a

MANAGING URGES AND CRAVINGS

- Distraction
- Imagery
  - Imagining negative consequences of addictive behavior
  - Imagining positive consequences of successful recovery
  - Imagery rehearsal
- Identifying alternative behaviors
- Coping cards
- Advantages–disadvantages analysis

REPAIRING EXISTING CLOSE RELATIONSHIPS

- Participation in shared activities
- Effective communication skills
  - Verbal communication skills
  - Nonverbal communication skills
  - Active listening

DEVELOPING HEALTHY NEW RELATIONSHIPS

- Meeting new people
- Effective communication skills
  - Verbal communication skills
  - Nonverbal communication skills
  - Active listening

MANAGING UNPLEASANT EMOTIONS

- Applying the cognitive strategies described in Chapter 7
- Activity monitoring and scheduling
- Controlled breathing and muscle relaxation

PROBLEM SOLVING

- Identifying and prioritizing problems
- Brainstorming potential solutions
- Evaluating potential solutions
- Implementing a solution
- Evaluating the solution

LEADING A HEALTHY LIFESTYLE

- Psychoeducation about [insert name of specific lifestyle habit]
- Monitoring of [insert name of specific lifestyle habit]
- Making behavioral adjustments in order to achieve [insert name of specific lifestyle habit]
  - Eating regular and nutritious meals
  - Keeping a regular sleep schedule
  - Adhering to medical and mental health treatment programs

FIGURE 8.1. CTAG coping skills.

goal-directed activity such as cleaning the house or washing the car. It can be an inspirational activity such as reading a poem, a favorite quote, or a religious text. Patients have license to be quite creative when identifying effective distraction strategies.

Sometimes patients have difficulty identifying distraction strategies that would be helpful, as they have not had a great deal of experience in using them in the past. Facilitators might have a list of typical distraction activities prepared in advance, and group members who have successfully used distraction in the past might be able to help new members identify ways to adapt the strategies in their own lives. Such a list could be one that is generated by the facilitators on the basis of their clinical experience, or one that has been published in other treatment manuals such as Linehan's (1993) *Skills Training Manual for Borderline Personality Disorder* or Muñoz, Ippen, Rao, Le, and Dwyer's (2000) *Manual for Group Cognitive-Behavioral Therapy of Depression: A Reality Management Approach* (Activities Module, Participant Manual, pp. 55–56). Facilitators can even work collaboratively with group members during session to construct a list of distraction strategies that is personalized for the group.

In our experience, each group member is unique in that there are particular distraction strategies that work well for one person, but not necessarily for another person. When distraction is the coping skill of focus, facilitators guide group members in identifying the particular distraction exercises that would be most useful to them and that they can use in the time before the next session. Facilitators also make explicit that distraction is not a long-term solution for managing addictive behavior. Instead, distraction should be viewed as a short-term strategy to survive intense urges and cravings, which contrasts with changes in unhelpful beliefs and the development of a healthy lifestyle that are expected to reduce urges and cravings in the long run.

Imagery

As mentioned in the previous section, imagery can be used as a distraction technique, in that group members can vividly imagine pleasant scenes when faced with an urge or craving. However, imagery is a versatile strategy that can be used for several other purposes, such as reminding oneself of the negative consequences of engaging in addictive behavior, acknowledging the positive consequences of not engaging in addictive behavior, or rehearsing the coping skills learned in CTAGs. In the former two cases, it would be considered another avenue for stimulus control. In the latter case, imagery would serve as a vehicle to achieve counterconditioning, or substituting an unhealthy cognitive or behavioral response for a healthy one. Consider the following vignette:

FACILITATOR 1: Many group members over the years have found it helpful to have a vision of the negative consequences that could occur as a result of continuing to engage in their addictive behavior. When they experience urges and craving, they call up this vision and run it through their minds, almost like a movie. As they say in AA, "Play the tape through."

DAVE: (looking skeptical)

FACILITATOR 2: Dave, your facial expression suggests that you don't buy this.

DAVE: No, I don't at all. I don't know how something like this could possibly work when I have been drinking and using drugs for the majority of my life. It's like my body needs them or something.

FACILITATOR 1: I appreciate your candor, Dave. Has anyone else had similar doubts?

ELLEN: Depending on the day, I have doubts about all of these strategies, Dave. I guess I just focus on the fact that any strategy is better than no strategy.

BRIAN: I agree with Ellen. And I also know where you're coming from. I've had a hard time really using this stuff when I'm outside of group. So, I think it's important for all of us to really practice.

FACILITATOR 1: That's a good point, Brian. Let's consider for a minute how envisioning a negative consequence might work, so that the reasoning behind it is clear. Does anyone have any ideas?

ALLISON: I guess it could distract you?

FACILITATOR 1: That's right, on a very basic level it turns your attention away from the craving. Does anyone else have any ideas?

MICHAEL: Well, I've actually done this. You had us do this in group a few months ago. What I found is that it only kind of worked at first, but I kept with it, and it started to work better as time went on.

FACILITATOR 1: Michael has made an important point that I'd like to emphasize. If you keep at it, over time your mind will start associating the craving with negative consequences rather than your addiction. But it takes time for that association to develop.

ELLEN: I also think that doing this could just make you stop and think about what you are doing, rather than just diving in and eating a pint of ice cream without thinking about it.

FACILITATOR 2: This is another important point. Having a negative image of the sequence of negative consequences will help to delay gratification and will force you to think through your decision before you decide to engage in the addictive behavior. Michael, would you be willing to share with the group the image of negative consequences that you use when you experience urges and cravings?

MICHAEL: OK. I just picture my wife's face when she's found out that I've been with another woman.

FACILITATOR 2: Is that the extent of your image?

MICHAEL: No, like you taught us, it's important to think about both the short-term and long-term consequences. So then I picture her screaming and crying, saying that she knew I would never change. (*speaking more softly*) And then I picture her packing up a suitcase, taking the kids, and saying she is leaving me.

FACILITATOR 1: (*gently*) Is that an effective strategy in preventing you from acting upon your urges?

MICHAEL: Yeah, it sure is. It's a cold hard fact that I could lose everything if I don't get this under control.

Just as imagery can be used to develop a sequence of negative consequences associated with addictive behavior, it can also be used to elaborate upon the positive consequences of refraining from engaging in addictive behavior. Consider the following vignette, in which the facilitators help Allison to elaborate upon her "snapshot" of being in the doctor's office and getting a "clean bill of health":

FACILITATOR 1: (*after educating the group on the usefulness of developing a sequence of images of positive consequences*) Allison, I think we can take your image of getting a clean bill of health even further so that you can really focus on the positive consequences of not smoking next time you get an urge. Can you think of other consequences of not giving into the urge?

ALLISON: Well, it sounds like something little, but one thing I've always wanted to do is go out with some of the girls after work. They do this about once a week. I never went with them because I always worried that I'd want to smoke if I was out, and then it would be embarrassing to have to get up and go outside. That always made me feel bad because I don't have a lot of support outside of my family, and I think I'd really get along with these girls if I spent some time with them outside of work.

FACILITATOR 2: So how would this translate into an image of the positive consequences of not smoking?

ALLISON: Well, I guess I would picture myself going out with them after work, laughing and enjoying ourselves, and maybe even becoming good friends.

FACILITATOR 2: Excellent. So your personal sequence of positive consequences associated with not smoking starts with an image of getting a clean bill of health from the doctor, and then moving into a social setting where you're doing things and developing relationships that smoking previously prevented you from pursing. Are there any other positive consequences, perhaps some that are even longer-term, that you could add to this?

ALLISON: (*more softly*) You know, after smoking for so long, I actually wasn't sure that I'd live long enough to see my grandchildren grow up. My daughter has a little girl who is only a baby, and my other children haven't had kids yet. Maybe I have something to live for now.

ELLEN: That is really lovely, Allison. I think that's the perfect vision of positive consequences.

ALLISON: (*smiling gratefully*)

FACILITATOR 1: (*to the group*) Michael and Allison have provided great examples of how to be creative in constructing these images of positive and negative consequences. Michael's image focuses primarily on one night and the events that would occur if his wife found out that he was into pornography again. In contrast, Allison's image contains a series of snapshots that go further and further out in time, all the way to several years from now when she is healthy and able to spend time with her grandchildren.

Another way imagery can be effective is for group members to imagine themselves implementing the coping skills learned in the CTAG, a strategy briefly introduced in Chapter 7, called *imagery rehearsal* (A. T. Beck et al., 1993). It is helpful for facilitators to take time in session to guide group members as they go through this exercise, as doing this helps to solidify the image so that it is readily accessible when group members experience urges and cravings in their daily lives. When these images are activated during urges and cravings, they can remind group members of how to apply their coping skills. Without these images, group members might be unable to capitalize on the skills because of feeling overwhelmed, not knowing where to start, or forgetting what they learned due to the intensity of the cravings. Sometimes group members express concern that they will not be able to implement the coping skills even after bringing up such an image. In these instances, it is helpful to have patients imagine themselves *being successful* in using the coping skills so that the image is associated with a sense of mastery and self-efficacy.

Identifying Alternative Behaviors

Functional analysis is a behavioral strategy to understand why a behavior is maintained over time (cf. Higgins, Sigmon, & Heil, 2008; McCrady, 2008). As part of a functional analysis, the positive consequences that follow the behavior (and that serve to maintain the behavior) are enumerated. In other words, functional analysis helps to identify the underlying *function* or *purpose* of the behavior. People engage in addictive behavior for a number of reasons—to seek excitement, to relieve anxiety, to fill a void, to decrease boredom, and so on. It can be helpful for facilitators to guide group members in identifying the function underlying their addictive behaviors and use that information to identify alternative, healthier ways to obtain those reinforcers (cf. L. C. Sobell & Sobell, 2011). This process achieves self-liberation, in that group members become aware of alternative choices to their addictive behavior. It also achieves counterconditioning because group members substitute healthier behaviors for addictive behaviors.

Consider the vignette with Dave from Chapter 7. With the help of the facilitators, it was determined that going to the bar was a way of relieving the significant distress he experienced when his girlfriend told him that she thought she was pregnant. Instead of evaluating Dave's thoughts about the situation and linking them to his underlying belief about being trapped, the facilitators also could have helped him to understand what function the drinking would serve and how he could get his needs met in a different way:

> FACILITATOR 2: So you were experiencing a range of intense emotions, and the way you chose to cope with them, watching a race on TV, wasn't effective. And then you had the thought, "Screw it. I might as well go get drunk because I'm not going to have fun in about 7 months."
>
> DAVE: That's about the size of it.
>
> FACILITATOR 2: Why drink in this situation, Dave?
>
> DAVE: I don't get what you mean. Because I couldn't deal with it anymore!
>
> FACILITATOR 2: OK, let me put it another way, what did drinking *do* for you in this situation?
>
> DAVE: It took my mind off of it. So I didn't have to think about it anymore.
>
> BRIAN: Kind of like an escape?

DAVE: Yeah, you could put it like that.

MICHAEL: I think we all want to escape our stress or misery at some time or another. I don't blame you, Dave.

FACILITATOR 1: Dave, it's understandable that you would want a break, an escape. It sounds like that news really caught you off guard and triggered a lot of unpleasant images and emotions in you. But what we're wondering is whether there was a way to achieve the same goal—the break, or the escape—without going to the bar and getting drunk.

DAVE: I have no idea.

FACILITATOR 1: So every time you need a break, do you go to the bar and get drunk?

DAVE: (*sheepishly*) A lot of the time, I guess.

FACILITATOR 1: But not all the time?

DAVE: No, not all the time.

ALLISON: So what else do you do?

DAVE: I go out to my friend's garage, where I keep an old truck I'm working on. It doesn't run yet. But I keep getting old parts and messing around with it.

FACILITATOR 1: And that's an escape for you?

DAVE: Yeah. I can work on it for hours.

FACILITATOR 2: Next time you feel like you want a break, like you want to escape, could you accomplish that by going and working on your truck instead of going to a bar and getting drunk?

DAVE: Actually, I think I could. Sometimes when that happens I just want to be alone, and you know how bars are. You can't really be alone there. Sometimes people there really bug me.

Unlike most instances in which the facilitators attempt to implement an intervention with Dave, this one went surprisingly smoothly because Dave was readily able to identify another activity that could give him a temporary escape. Many group members are not so easily convinced that another activity could substitute for the addictive behavior and achieve the same goal. In these cases, it is helpful to devise a behavioral experiment in order to test the belief that the substitute activity will not achieve its goal. In Ellen's case, the facilitators helped her to determine that the function of eating was to give her some of the satisfaction she was missing in her life. After brainstorming some activities that also might provide a sense of satisfaction, Ellen settled on quilting, an activity that had won her awards at craft fairs in the past but that she had largely abandoned as her depression worsened. However, Ellen was far from convinced that it would give her as much satisfaction as eating would:

ELLEN: I don't know, I really just don't have the energy right now to start a new project.

MICHAEL: That's the depression talking, Ellen. Trust me, I've been there in the past.

ELLEN: I know, Michael, I know. You're so right. But I'm stuck in a rut, and I can't seem to get out.

FACILITATOR 1: I'll tell you what. What if we were to conduct an experiment? Next time you experience a strong sense that something is missing from your life, would you be willing to try quilting instead of eating to get that sense of satisfaction?

ELLEN: I'd like to, but I think it's easier said than done.

FACILITATOR 1: I understand, you don't have a lot of energy right now. What I think might help would be objective evidence that this strategy is helpful. Next time you experience a strong sense that something is missing from your life, rate that degree to which you experience dissatisfaction with your life on a 0–10 scale. Then try quilting for a bit, and rate your level of dissatisfaction again. If you try this a few times, and the rating doesn't go down, then you'll know this strategy doesn't work well in addressing this problem, and I won't suggest it to you again. But what if the rating *does* go down?

ELLEN: (*pausing*) I guess then I'd know I have a good coping strategy to use, since nothing really has worked so far.

Because Ellen was experiencing significant symptoms of depression, it was important for the facilitators to do everything possible to ensure that the strategy could be implemented successfully. The facilitators suspected that relying on the vague act of "quilting" might be overwhelming for Ellen in the moment, when she is overcome with sadness associated with life dissatisfaction. The facilitators enlisted the other group members to identify ways to increase the likelihood that Ellen could successfully use quilting as a strategy to manage urges and cravings to overeat:

FACILITATOR 1: In my experience, it's usually best to have a specific plan in place for the use of other activities to meet the same need as your addiction. In the moment, the urges and cravings can be experienced as so overwhelming that it is difficult to get started on something else unless it is laid out for you. Has anyone had that experience?

BRIAN: I know exactly what you mean. I have the best laid plans, and then, boom, next thing I know, I'm at the casino.

ALLISON: Ellen, do you have any specific project that you're working on?

ELLEN: No, not really. I'm not even sure where I would start.

FACILITATOR 1: That's very important to know, Ellen. If you don't know where to start now, it will be very difficult to use this coping strategy when you are in distress and experiencing urges and cravings. Maybe the group can help you to develop a plan?

(*Group members nod their heads.*)

ALLISON: What if you were to decide on a project in advance and get everything you need for it, so that it is right there for you?

ELLEN: That could work. My niece just had a baby, and I'd love to make a quilt for him.

MICHAEL: I wonder if you should start the project a little bit first, before you really need to rely on it to resist eating. That way, you might have less trouble getting started.

ELLEN: I think that's a great idea. One of my biggest problems is getting started with anything other than eating.

FACILITATOR 2: Excellent suggestions. Ellen, when might you go out and get the supplies you need?

ELLEN: It sounds like I better do this sooner rather than later, before I lose momentum. I'll stop at my favorite craft store on the way home from group.

Coping Cards

As stated in Chapter 7, coping cards contain reminders of cognitive and behavioral strategies that are useful in managing mood, accomplishing a goal, or responding to a difficult situation. Patients often report that they have difficulty thinking of anything other than engaging in their addictive behavior when they experience urges and cravings. Thus, coping cards are important aids for group members to consult during these times to be reminded of ways they can actively deal with urges and cravings, the positive consequences of successfully managing them, and the consequences for succumbing to them.

Coping cards for managing urges and cravings can take many forms and can summarize any of the strategies described in this book. For example, group members might write a facilitating thought that would give them permission to engage in addictive behavior on one side of the card and an alternative response on the other side of the card. They might list distraction techniques that they had successfully used in the past. They might provide a detailed description of their image of positive consequences of not engaging in the addictive behavior or the image of the negative consequences of slipping. Or they might simply list a host of reasons why they should not give in to the urges and cravings. Quite simply, coping cards can contain any types of reminders for patients to respond rationally in times of distress, when they might forget the cognitive and behavioral interventions discussed in the CTAG. Because of their versatility, they can be used to achieve many of the processes of change included in the TTM (Prochaska & DiClemente, 2005).

Advantages–Disadvantages Analysis

When group members struggling with addictions find themselves alone, down, and experiencing a craving, it is quite a temptation to give up and engage in the addictive behavior. In other instances, group members do not intentionally set out to engage in addictive behavior, but they return to familiar places where they once engaged in addictive behavior in order to run into familiar faces (i.e., "seemingly irrelevant decisions"; Monti et al., 2002; Rotgers & Nguyen, 2006). An agreed-upon tenet among addictions treatment professionals, regardless of their orientation, is that returning to such a "hangout" significantly increases a person's vulnerability for a slip or lapse (e.g., Shiffman, Paty, Gnys, Kassel, & Hickcox, 1996). Thus, facilitators can use cognitive and behavioral strategies to reduce the likelihood that group members will seek out these former hangouts or otherwise put themselves in a position in which they will engage in addictive behavior.

A particularly useful cognitive therapy strategy to introduce in these situations is the *advantages–disadvantages analysis*. This technique is sometimes referred to as decisional balance (Rotgers & Nguyen, 2006; L. C. Sobell & Sobell, 2011), or weighing pros and cons (e.g., Velasquez, Maurer, Crouch, & DiClemente, 2001). Using a whiteboard, facilitators can draw a 2×2 quadrant with four cells such that the advantages and disadvantages of engaging in addictive behavior or in returning to the hangout and of not engaging in addictive behavior or staying away from the hangout are listed. They invite group members to supply items for each of the four quadrants, recording them along the way and subsequently encouraging group members to draw conclusions on the basis of their responses. The advantages–disadvantages analysis can achieve both self- and environmental reevaluation, as it allows group members the space to carefully evaluate the impact of problematic behavior on themselves, others, and their circumstances. This strategy is illustrated nicely with Dave, who, in a session that occurred a few months into his participation in the CTAG, had just expressed that he wanted to "catch up with the guys" who hang out at a bar that is near to his home:

> FACILITATOR 1: Dave, what I'm hearing is that you'd like to get out of the house and spend some time with your old friends.
>
> DAVE: Yeah. All I do now is work and stay at home with my girlfriend. I'm not even that interested in drinking, I just want to shoot some pool, see the guys, maybe catch a race on TV.
>
> MICHAEL: That sounds like a dangerous situation to me. Is there any way you can spend time with friends in a setting where there is no alcohol?
>
> DAVE: I know what you're thinking, that I'll drink just because I'm in a bar. But I've been in group now for 3 months, and haven't had a beer in a week and a half! I just want to play pool, man.
>
> FACILITATOR 1: Well, let's look at this systematically and then decide. I'd like to do an advantages–disadvantages analysis with you. We can invite the group to help if you'd like. Are you game?
>
> DAVE: (sighing) Fine!
>
> FACILITATOR 2: (drawing four quadrants on the whiteboard) Let's start with this box here on the upper left side. What are the advantages of going to the bar tonight?
>
> DAVE: Lots of them. I get to play pool, which I haven't done in a long time. I get to catch up with the guys. I get to get away from my girlfriend for a while. I don't know, just generally have fun.
>
> FACILITATOR 2: (writing Dave's advantages) Now what are the disadvantages of going to the bar?
>
> DAVE: Well, I don't think this will be a problem, but I suppose you would say that there will be alcohol there.
>
> FACILITATOR 2: And why is that a disadvantage?
>
> DAVE: It's not; like I said, I can handle it.
>
> FACILITATOR 1: Let's get some help from the rest of the group. Why might the fact that alcohol is present in Dave's choice of hangout be problematic?
>
> BRIAN: You're going to want to drink, man. I can guarantee it. It's still too soon for you.
>
> ELLEN: I was going to say that too. And another thing, if you keep going back to the same people who drink and use drugs, you'll

never have an opportunity to meet new people who are better for you.

ALLISON: Plus, you're just doing the same old thing again—going to the bar when things get stressful at home. You're not using all of the skills we've talked about in group to work on things with your girlfriend.

(*Group goes on to help Dave complete the advantages and disadvantages of staying away from the bar.*)

FACILITATOR 1: This is quite a list. After reviewing these advantages and disadvantages, Dave, what do you think now about going to the bar?

DAVE: I'd still like to go to play pool, and I still think I can handle it.... (*trailing off, suggesting there is more to his thought on the subject*)

FACILITATOR 1: ... and?

DAVE: (*reluctantly*) I guess there's more to it, though. I guess, deep down, I know that the guys I'll see at the bar are bad news for me. And going to the bar won't make things any better at home, probably a lot worse.

BRIAN: It's tough. Take it from me, I've gone to the casino so many times, thinking I could handle just spending $25 or $50. Never once did I get out of there without spending a whole lot more.

REPAIRING EXISTING CLOSE RELATIONSHIPS

Recall that, in Chapter 2, we introduced a weak social support network as a distal vulnerability factor for addictive behavior. Research shows that a strong social support network is highly predictive of recovery, whereas weak social support is highly predictive of relapse (e.g., Chen, 2010; Palmer, Murphy, Piselli, & Ball, 2009). In addition, research has found that cognitive behavioral treatment that includes an interpersonal component (i.e., development of skills to improve relationships) is associated with a greater reduction in alcohol use than cognitive behavioral treatment that focuses only on mood management (Monti et al., 1990). Thus, the interpersonal environment of the person struggling with addictions can play a crucial role in his or her recovery.

It is no secret that the close relationships of people who struggle with addictions often have suffered tremendously because of the addictive behavior (Rotgers & Nguyen, 2006). It is not uncommon for patients with addictions to have cheated on, lied to, or stolen from some of their closest family members and friends. Empirical research shows that some addictive behaviors, such as alcohol addiction, are associated with negative marital interaction patterns and even marital violence (Marshal, 2003). When patients enter treatment, family members and friends are often in the precarious position of wanting to support them through the treatment process but of feeling a need to be on guard for "getting burned." Not surprisingly, family members and friends often lack trust, harbor feelings of anger and resentment, and quickly call patients to task when there is even the slightest indication of a slip. Group members, who are already prone to mood swings as they are learning to manage urges and cravings, often feel frustrated and irritated at the perceived lack of support of those in their support network.

Although trust can be rebuilt in many ways, the "bottom line" is that it does not happen overnight and takes time. Cognitive strategies are usually used in conjunction with the relationship-building strategies described in this section, as some group members report cognitions that could thwart their efforts (e.g., "There's no use in trying"). In addition, it is important for group members to formulate realistic expectations about the fact that rebuilding relationships takes time and that they likely will not see a direct correspondence between the efforts they put into it and the reception of others, at least in the beginning. Cognitive strategies are crucial in ensuring that group members do not become discouraged if they do not see tangible benefits from their efforts and in accepting the uncertainty about the status of their relationships.

Each of the group members described in this book has specific deficits in his or her close relationships. Ellen, for example, has distant and unsupportive relationships with the small number of people in her family, and she could benefit from strategies to develop stronger familial relationships. Dave has frequent arguments with his live-in girlfriend and is estranged from his father, and he could benefit from strategies to communicate effectively and manage conflict. Allison's husband and mother-in-law continue to smoke in her presence, and she could benefit from strategies to assert her wishes that they not smoke in the house and negotiate compromises about their smoking. Michael's wife opted to remain in the marriage but admits she does not trust him, which has created tension in their relationship and is a source of frustration. Brian's wife is contemplating divorcing him because he has compromised their future by spending nearly all of their assets on gambling. Both Michael and Brian could benefit from strategies to tolerate their spouses' anger and ambivalence and to persist in engaging in adaptive behaviors that will restore trust.

In this section, we describe two common relationship-building strategies that have been useful for previous CTAG members: (1) participation in shared activities, and (2) development of effective communication skills. Many of these skills simultaneously capitalize on several processes of change. At a basic level, they achieve counterconditioning because group members replace unhealthy relationship behaviors with healthy ones. They also achieve stimulus control because successful acquisition of these skills has the potential to manage triggers (e.g., relationship conflict) that could serve as a trigger for engaging in addictive behavior. However, they also harness another process of change—helping relationships—because, as close relationships are repaired, group members will be able to garner support for their continued work on managing their addiction.

Participation in Shared Activities

CTAG members often remark that they have to learn an entirely new way of relating to and engaging with family members and friends now that they are no longer actively addicted. We have found it helpful for group members to *participate in shared activities* with these individuals. Through these shared activities, group members can reacquaint themselves with their family members and friends without the veil of the addiction. Participation in activities of mutual interest will help to reestablish the bond or connection that was once there. Repeated engagement in these activities will help family members and friends to slowly develop confidence that the group member can function well without engaging in addictive behavior and has developed skills to prevent relapse. Additionally, engaging in shared activities is a way of experiencing pleasure, which is an important antidote against depression.

Consider the case of Dave. In previous CTAGs, he had expressed anger at his father for "being a drunk" throughout Dave's childhood and admitted that he rarely talks to his father because of his resentment. The group learned that Dave's father has been sober for over 5 years, and many members commented about the possibility of his father being a support for Dave as he goes through recovery. For homework, Dave agreed (reluctantly!) to ask his father to help him work on his truck in order to engage in a shared experience as a way to rebuild their relationship. In this vignette, he reports back to the group:

> FACILITATOR 1: Last week we talked about ways to enhance our close relationships, relationships with family and friends. Each of you made the commitment to initiate one shared activity with a family member or friend with whom your relationship is strained because of your addiction. I'm curious about how that went for you.
>
> (*Group pauses.*)

ALLISON: I could go, but I have to admit, Dave, I'm dying to know what happened in your situation. Did you call your father?

DAVE: Yeah. Believe it or not, I did it. (*trying to suppress a smile*)

ALLISON: Wow, that's great! What happened.

DAVE: Well ... you probably remember that I wasn't really into this idea. I actually wasn't even going to do it. There's just too much bad blood there between us.

FACILITATOR 2: So what changed?

DAVE: (*laughing*) I ran into him at the gas station. I couldn't believe it! I said, "Just my luck that I would have to run into him *this* week when that was my homework assignment." (*Group erupts in laugher.*) So I was like, "What the hell, I might as well go the whole nine yards and ask him."

MICHAEL: What did you say?

DAVE: I just told him I was working on the truck and that I got stuck with something, which really is true. And my dad had been a mechanic for a long time, so I knew he'd know how to fix it.

MICHAEL: And what did he say?

DAVE: He seemed really surprised. At first I wasn't sure he'd say yes, since we've fought pretty hard the last few times we've seen each other. But he came over.

FACILITATOR 2: And how did it go?

DAVE: It was seriously the first time in years, longer than I can remember, where we were together and both of us were sober and we weren't getting on each other's nerves.

ELLEN: Did you fix the truck?

DAVE: Yeah, we fixed the truck. Then after that we got something to eat. (*Group nods in approval and encouragement.*)

MICHAEL: Did you guys talk about your drinking and his drinking?

DAVE: No, we didn't get that far. I didn't want to ruin it, since we were actually getting along. (*more softly*) I actually felt like I had a father for once, and I just wanted to keep it like that for a minute, you know, like appreciate it.

FACILITATOR 1: What did you learn from all of this?

DAVE: You know, I learned things about him that I never knew. Like that he tried to go to school at the community college when I was a kid, in order to get a degree and move us out of the trailer park, but that he just couldn't cut it, with paying for school and having to work at the same time. And all this time I thought he was just a lazy bastard who didn't give a shit if he lived in the trailer park for the rest of his life.

FACILITATOR 1: Dave, I can't tell you how happy I am for you that you and your father made this important step in repairing your relationship. And for the rest of you, this is a good example of how engaging in a shared activity that both people enjoy, like working on the truck, can facilitate a connection and even lead to realizations about the other person that you never thought possible. How do you think this might help you overcome your addiction?

DAVE: Maybe he does understand more than I think he does. Maybe I can talk to him about ideas of ways to start taking my life in a different direction.

At times, group members balk at this strategy for relationship building. Some members view it is as simplistic and self-evident; others view it as "easier said than done" and avoid initiating these activities with others because of the expectation of rejection. For the former type of group member, it is important that facilitators provide a clear rationale for the activity, so that he or she has a sound understanding of the manner in which addressing this distal background factor will help with his or her recovery. For the latter type of group member, facilitators can use cognitive strategies to evaluate the idea that he or she will be rejected when initiating activities with family members and friends. For example, the facilitators might encourage the group member to make a realistic estimation of the worst thing that might happen or to evaluate whether rejection of the offer to engage in a particular activity is equal to an overall rejection of the group member as a person.

Effective Communication Skills

It is not uncommon for patients with addictions to lack the skills necessary to communicate effectively with close others, either to manage conflict or to be assertive in expressing their needs. After they recover from their addiction, many patients realize that their addictive behavior had a profound effect on the style in which they approached these interactions. Some patients are passive; they require cognitive interventions to modify the belief that they do not have a right to express their opinion and behavioral skills to develop assertiveness. In contrast, other patients are aggressive; they require cognitive interventions to reduce their sense of entitlement and behavioral skills to develop negotiating and listening skills. Others are somewhere in between, but have gotten "stuck" in problematic communication patterns with one or more close others and require interventions to establish more adaptive ways of interacting. There are three main areas of communication skills training that are often covered in CTAGs—verbal communication, nonverbal communication, and active listening. Figure 8.2 lists a number of specific skills in these three main areas that can assume the focus in any one session. Practice of these communication skills allows for many of Yalom and Leszcz's (2005) therapeutic factors to emerge, including the imparting of information, imitative behavior, development of socializing techniques, and interpersonal learning.

Facilitators make the judgment of the particular communication skill or skills on which to focus using (1) information obtained during

---

VERBAL COMMUNICATION

- Using "I" language and taking ownership of opinions
- Providing a clear rationale for requests
- Focusing on the main idea without getting derailed
- Balancing positives and negatives
- Commenting on the communication process when there is a "stuck" point
- Refraining from insults, accusations, and sarcasm
- Calming down before saying something in anger or frustration
- Conversing about appropriate topics
- Being willing to compromise
- Refraining from apologizing for making requests, having an opinion, or saying "no"

NONVERBAL COMMUNICATION

- Making appropriate eye contact
- Making appropriate facial expressions
- Nodding and making gestures at appropriate times
- Assuming an open (vs. closed) and a relaxed, upright posture
- Maintaining an appropriate amount of personal space
- Refraining from engaging in nervous habits (e.g., tapping fingers, twisting hair)
- Using an appropriate tone of voice and rate of speaking

ACTIVE LISTENING

- Refraining from interrupting before the other person has finished
- Summarizing or paraphrasing what the other has said
- Asking for clarification before responding
- Using nonverbal behavior to communicate interest

FIGURE 8.2. Examples of effective communication skills. Many of these communication skills are described in more length in Monti et al. (2002) and Paterson (2000).

the introductions, particularly when group members comment on "other issues" that have been problematic for them; and (2) observations of the communication style of group members across several sessions. They then use a combination of didactic instruction, demonstration in front of the group with one group member, and role plays in pairs in order to illustrate the manner in which the skill(s) can be implemented in particular situations. It is often helpful to approach these skills from an inquisitive standpoint, asking group members to describe how they would feel and react in situations in which maladaptive versus adaptive skills are being used by another person. Consider the case of Allison, who is having difficulty negotiating rules about smoking in the house with her husband and mother-in-law:

> ALLISON: It's just so frustrating! During the day, I feel like I've made progress because I'm at work, focused on what I'm doing, and rarely having a craving. But then I come home to a smoke-filled house, and I go back to square one.
>
> ELLEN: Have you told your husband and mother-in-law how you feel?
>
> ALLISON: I sure have. They basically say that they shouldn't have to suffer just because I'm the one with the problem.
>
> ELLEN: You're kidding me! That's awful!
>
> FACILITATOR 2: Exactly how did you communicate your concerns? What did you say?
>
> ALLISON: (*pausing, thinking*) I said that I wish they would stop smoking in front of me, that it is inconsiderate given that I have serious health problems because of smoking.
>
> FACILITATOR 2: Allison, would you mind role-playing this with me in front of the group so we can get an even better handle on what's happening when you have these interactions with your husband and mother-in-law?
>
> ALLISON: (*reluctantly*) Well, OK.
>
> FACILITATOR 2: Great. You play you, and I'll play your husband. I'd like you to say, as accurately as possible, what you've said in previous situations like this. OK?
>
> ALLISON: (*nodding*)
>
> FACILITATOR 2: Why don't we start with you walking in the kitchen and seeing the two of them smoking?
>
> ALLISON: (*timidly*) Could you go outside to smoke? I told you before I can't have smoke in the house.

FACILITATOR 2: Well, I've had a hard day and could really use a smoke. Why don't *you* go somewhere else if the smoke is bothering you?

ALLISON: Because this is my house too! And besides, I can't avoid the kitchen forever.

FACILITATOR 2: Well, I'm not going to pay the price for your health problems.

ALLISON: (*Seems exasperated and mutters, "See? What an asshole!"*)

FACILITATOR 2: Is that how it ends, Allison? With you muttering "asshole"?

ALLISON: Sometimes. But more often than not, I'm so angry and frustrated and hurt all at once that I think I'll probably burst out crying if I open my mouth again.

FACILITATOR 1: So what do you do?

ALLISON: Sometimes I go in the bedroom and just cry. Or sometimes I go in the living room and watch TV. But we have a small place, so I can still smell the smoke.

FACILITATOR 1: What happens when you are face-to-face with your husband again? Do you talk about it more?

ALLISON: No, we pretty much just give each other the cold shoulder. And there have been a lot of cold shoulders these days.

MICHAEL: Man, that does not sound fun at all.

ALLISON: No, it isn't. It's getting to the point where I'm uncomfortable in my own home.

On the basis of this information, the facilitators could choose to focus on one of any number of communication skills. For example, Allison's request is clear, but her communication style could be improved by providing a more compelling rationale for her request (e.g., the severity of her health problems, the extent to which she struggles with having smoke in the house, the precise doctor's orders). It is possible that providing such information would help her husband better understand the reasons for and depth of her concerns. Thus, the facilitators could educate the group about the usefulness of including a rationale with a request and have the group help Allison to formulate a compelling rationale that might accompany her request. In addition, Allison drops the conversation after her husband tells her he won't pay the price for her health problems. Here, the facilitators might introduce the concept of the "broken record," in which an individual repeatedly communicates his or her main point without getting derailed (e.g., Paterson, 2000). When people use the "broken record," they communicate that they have an important point they want to be known and that they will not be derailed by another person's resistance or attempt to change the topic of conversation. Allison also uses the term *asshole*, which likely increases her husband's resistance to making any concessions about smoking. This example can illustrate an important point about verbal communication—that insults, accusations, and sarcasm only make the quality of an interaction deteriorate. Finally, the facilitators might note the fact that Allison's husband and mother-in-law agreed to refrain from smoking in certain areas of the house, such as the living room. Although smoking in the kitchen has turned out to be problematic for Allison, the facilitators might encourage her to acknowledge the changes that *have* been made in order to balance out the new request.

In any of these interventions, facilitators can solicit assistance from the group to address Allison's issues, invite group members to provide examples of the communication skill from their own experience, or request descriptions of similar problems to provide another instance for the group to formulate an alternative verbal response. They also are aware of cognitions that have the potential to interfere with the successful application of effective coping skills and use the strategies described in Chapter 7 to reframe them.

At times, the group will focus its efforts on one or two of the effective communication skills, practicing ways to apply them to a range of situations involving close others. In other instances, group members all resonate with one common situation that has the potential to serve as a trigger for a slip, lapse, or emotional upset (e.g., being offered an opportunity to engage in addictive behavior, such as having a drink or going to a casino), and they apply a large number of the effective communication skills to negotiate this situation. Figure 8.3 lists a number of common situations that have been addressed in the CTAG, as well as in other cognitive behavioral

---

- Refusing an opportunity to engage in addictive behavior
- Responding to close others who are excessively vigilant for signs of a slip or relapse
- Responding to close others who make inquiries about a slip or relapse
- Responding to close others' anger about the consequences of the group member's addictive behavior
- Responding to criticisms made by close others
- Giving criticism to close others
- Saying "no" to close others

FIGURE 8.3. Situations requiring practice of effective communication skills. Many of these situations are referenced in Monti et al. (2002) and Rotgers and Nguyen (2006).

treatments for managing addictive behavior (e.g., Monti et al., 2002; Rotgers & Nguyen, 2006). In fact, facilitators can come to group ahead of time with prepared scenarios that illustrate these common situations, and group members can practice the application of effective communication skills (cf. Monti et al., 2002).

DEVELOPING NEW HEALTHY RELATIONSHIPS

In addition to problems with their partner and family relationships, patients with addictions often realize that the majority of their social network continues to engage in addictive behavior, which undermines their attempt to recover (McCrady, 2008). When they spend time with these individuals, patients quickly find that they revert back to their former (and maladaptive) cognitive and behavioral tendencies. They are particularly vulnerable to slips and lapses under these circumstances. Thus, patients with addictions often find themselves in the position of having to build a brand new social network during their time of recovery. This is a tall order, particularly in light of the fact that these patients are accustomed to interacting with other people while they are engaging in addictive behavior (e.g., talking with others at bars while drinking) and that they are vulnerable to low mood and frustration.

When group members bring up feelings of loneliness and isolation during the introductions, the facilitators can focus on developing new healthy relationships during the body of the CTAG. We find that the focus on developing new healthy relationships takes on one of two main themes: (1) staying away from places where there is an opportunity to engage in addictive behaviors (e.g., bars, strip clubs), and (2) developing skills to initiate and nurture new relationships. The advantages–disadvantages analysis described earlier in this chapter is useful for staying away from former hangouts.

Many patients, whether or not they struggle with addictions, indicate that they do not know where to begin when faced with the challenge of meeting others and forming new relationships. They often have trouble identifying appropriate places to meet others, and they worry that they will not know what to say when they are beginning to get acquainted with others. Patients with addictions often raise concerns about whether others will want to pursue a relationship with them once they learn of their sordid pasts. Thus, the development of new relationships is a topic that is particularly engaging for most group members, and the group provides a forum for relationships among group members to strengthen because of the shared experience. This section considers two relevant topics: (1) identifying ways to meet new people, and (2) developing effective communication strategies for use in fledgling relationships. These strategies work through several processes of change. Specifically, they achieve social liberation, in that group members are actively creating an environment that allows them to make healthier choices. They achieve counterconditioning by replacing unhealthy behaviors with healthy behaviors, as well as stimulus control, because the development of new relationships is an antidote against loneliness, which could serve as a trigger for engaging in addictive behavior.

Meeting New People

We have found it helpful for group members to generate a list of ways to meet new people. Often, these lists comprise items such as get to know people at work, pursue an activity (e.g., join a local gym or sports team), go to a place of worship such as a church or synagogue, go to 12-step meetings, and become more involved with the community. Seasoned group members have the opportunity to share their successes with newer group members and identify particular approaches that work well in fostering new relationships in appropriate settings. A logical homework assignment is for each group member to attempt one item on the list in the upcoming week.

It is also important to integrate cognitive strategies as group members begin to initiate and nurture new relationships. Some group members become discouraged when they perceive progress as being slow. In these cases, it is important for facilitators to help the group formulate realistic expectations for the pace at which most new relationships develop. In addition, many group members are interpersonally sensitive, especially at this vulnerable time in their life when they are trying to sustain recovery. It is not uncommon for some group members to interpret actions of others as rebuffs and rejections. Thus, facilitators can use cognitive strategies to evaluate the evidence that supports and refutes the perception of rejection; how bad, realistically, one rejection would be; and whether rejection by one individual equals rejection by everyone.

Effective Communication Skills

Effective communication skills not only are important in repairing close relationships that were damaged by group members' addictions, but they are also important in developing new relationships. Thus, all of the communication skills summarized in Figure 8.2 can be applied to the development of new relationships. Discussion of these skills might take place in the context of concerns expressed by group members that are specific to developing new relationships. For example, some group members express concern that they do not know how to make "small talk" when they are free of the influence of alcohol or drugs. Other group members are concerned about being "out of practice" because their addiction had consumed so much time in their lives, leaving them little opportunity to socialize with others. Still others worry that there will be a temptation to engage in addictive behavior (e.g., someone will offer them a drink) and that they do not know how to refuse. Consider this vignette with Allison, when she was describing anxiety about an upcoming happy hour with her female coworkers:

ALLISON: I can't believe they asked me to go! But I'm *really* nervous. I'll have nothing to talk about with them.

ELLEN: I think you're going to do fine. You're very personable with us, here in group.

DAVE: Come on! You'll be fine.

ALLISON: Yeah, but this is different. In group, we're all here for the same reason, more or less, and there's a structure to the group. We know what to expect. I don't have any clue what to expect at the happy hour.

FACILITATOR 1: Might it be beneficial to take some time for the group to consider effective approaches to making "small talk" with a new group of people?

ALLISON: Oh yes, definitely.

ELLEN: I can use that, too. I really need to get out of the house.

FACILITATOR 1: Let's think as a group for a moment. What approaches to making "small talk" have worked for you in the past?

MICHAEL: I have to make "small talk" all the time with my clients and other coworkers. I find that making sure you come across as pleasant is key. Then people really respond to you.

FACILITATOR 2: Great suggestion, Michael. Now let's think about what it means to come across pleasantly.

MICHAEL: Things like smiling. Making eye contact. Being interested in what the other person is saying.

FACILITATOR 2: (*writing these communication skills on a whiteboard as Michael speaks*)

BRIAN: I always try to ask the other person questions. Mostly it's because I don't want to talk about myself and my problems. But, it ends up working out because people really like to talk about themselves.

FACILITATOR 2: (*writing "ask questions about the other person" on the whiteboard*)

DAVE: Make jokes. That's what I do. It lightens up the mood.

ALLISON: Oh God, I don't know any jokes!

FACILITATOR 1: (*simultaneously reinforcing Dave's spontaneous contribution, as he does not make many, and translating the recommendation into a more helpful suggestion for Allison*) Dave's point is well taken—using humor is a way to engage others and keep the conversation light and interesting. I wonder, does it always have to be through jokes?

MICHAEL: No, not at all. It can be telling a funny story that happened to you, or just laughing along with the other people if someone else is telling a funny story.

FACILITATOR 1: Exactly. (*pausing*) What do you think of this list, Allison? The group has come up with quite a lot of suggestions.

ALLISON: They are really helpful, thank you, all of you. I'm just so nervous though....

FACILITATOR 1: Sometimes our thoughts can get in the way of the effective use of these skills. I wonder if we should think, in advance, about the type of thoughts that could get in the way and ways to overcome those thoughts?

(*Group members nod.*)

In this case, the facilitators went on to apply the cognitive strategies described in Chapter 7 to address unhelpful cognitions that might hinder the effective application of the communication skills identified in session. Subsequently, they encouraged the group members to think about the cognitive and behavioral strategies that they used to connect with the other group members when they first started attending the group and the manner in which those strategies could apply in other social settings.

Other group members describe instances in which they perceive that they opened up "too much" and overwhelmed those with whom they were interacting. Here, facilitators might lead a discussion on finding the appropriate balance between communicating honestly but also appropriately, commensurate with how well they know the person with whom they are interacting. There is no one skill, per se, that achieves this balance, and what might feel like a good balance for one group member might not feel like a good balance for another group member. Nevertheless, group members can share instances when they felt overwhelmed by interactions with others and identify specific behaviors by the person with whom they were interacting that were off-putting to them. The advantages–disadvantages analysis, described earlier in this chapter, could be applied to the decision as to whether to disclose certain information early on in new relationships.

MANAGING UNPLEASANT EMOTIONS

As has been stated on many occasions throughout this volume, patients with addictions are vulnerable to mood disturbance such as depression, guilt, anxiety, anger, loneliness, and boredom. Many patients with addictions have spent years coping with their mood problems by engaging in the addictive behavior (e.g., drinking alcohol to relieve anxiety). In addition to not having their primary coping tool available, these patients are also struggling with multiple issues in their lives that would exacerbate mood disturbance in almost anyone. Thus, it is not uncommon for the management of mood problems to assume a primary focus during sessions.

All of the strategies for managing addictive behaviors and their associated problems can be applied to managing mood. There is an extensive literature that describes strategies to modify automatic thoughts and beliefs associated with mood disturbance in general (e.g., J. S. Beck, 2005, 2011), depression (e.g., A. T. Beck, 1976; Padesky & Greenberger, 1995; Muñoz et al., 2000; Burns, 1999), anxiety (A. T. Beck & Emery, 2005; Bourne, 2010; Craske & Barlow, 2006), and anger (A. T. Beck, 1999; Reilly, Shopshire, Durazzo, & Campbell, 2002), all of which contain material relevant to managing mood in the context of CTAGs. Thought Records, coping cards, behavioral experiments, advantage–disadvantages analyses, and so on can be used to modify depressogenic, guilty, anxious, angry, and lonely thinking in the same way they can be used to modify anticipatory, relief-oriented, and facilitating cognitions about addictive behavior. In this section, we describe two additional strategies that can be useful in addressing mood disturbance: (1) activity monitoring and scheduling, and (2) controlled breathing and muscle relaxation. These strategies achieve counterconditioning because they have the potential to replace unhealthy behaviors (e.g., engaging in addictive behavior) with healthier coping skills, and they achieve stimulus control because they have the potential to reduce unpleasant emotion that can serve as a trigger for engaging in addictive behavior.

Activity Monitoring and Scheduling

Typical symptoms of depression include loss of interest and/or pleasure in activities that were once enjoyable, fatigue, and difficulty concentrating, all of which decrease patients' motivation to be active and engaged with their environment. Depressed patients often report that it takes all of their energy to function at a basic level (e.g., going to work, keeping appointments) and that they forgo other social and recreational activities. Not surprisingly, this sort of lifestyle leaves them little to look forward to in life and few outlets to experience pleasure, which further exacerbates their depressive symptoms. This, in turn, increases the likelihood of a lapse or a slip.

A common cognitive therapy strategy for such a clinical presentation is *activity monitoring and scheduling*. Activity monitoring helps the facilitators and group members to have an accurate view of the activities in which they are actually engaging. Group members are provided with grids to complete the activity monitoring exercise. The grid contains cells for all hours of the day over a 7-day period. Group members are instructed to record an event in each cell, even if they are sleeping. For each activity, they make two ratings on a 0–10 scale—the degree of *accomplishment* they get from the activity (0 = *no accomplishment*, 10 = *a great deal of accomplishment*), and the degree of *pleasure* they feel when they are doing the activity (0 = *no pleasure*, 10 = *a great deal of pleasure*). After facilitators gather information about the activities in which group members are engaging, they can work with group members to schedule new activities that provide a sense of accomplishment and/or pleasure. Form 8.1 (at the end of the chapter) displays an activity log that can be used for either activity monitoring or activity scheduling.

Figure 8.4 displays a sample from Ellen's activity log. Her activity log provides the facilitators with some important information. First, it appears that Ellen is engaging in very little goal-directed activity, which reduces the probability that she will experience accomplishment and pleasure from her environment. In addition, it appears that Ellen derives most of her pleasure from eating, which, of course, undermines her attempts to manage her overeating. The facilitators might address these points with Ellen by enlisting the group to help her to brainstorm meaningful activities that she can add into her daily routine. Second, it appears that Ellen's activities are mainly solitary in nature. Thus, the facilitators might help her to identify people who might have been in her social support network in the past and initiate contact with them, or identify activities outside of her apartment that would allow her the opportunity to interact with fresh faces. Third, Ellen's activity log suggests that she is sleeping approximately 12 hours a day, getting up in the late morning. This behavioral pattern limits the degree to which she actively engages in her environment. The facilitators can suggest activity scheduling as a way to work in pleasurable or meaningful activities in the morning, with the intention of improving Ellen's mood.

Even in the absence of depression, it can be helpful to focus a session on engagement in meaningful activities. Many patients with addictions realize that there is a void in their lives when they discontinue engaging in addictive behavior, as the addiction consumed the majority of their time and did not allow them to nurture other interests. Group members can use their time in session to identify meaningful activities that once seemed not to be options for them when they were actively engaged in their addiction, make a commitment to pursuing them, and even schedule time in their daily routines to ensure that they follow through (cf. Monti et al., 2002). In

	Day 1	Day 2	Day 3
7–8 A.M.	Sleep A = 1; P = 3	Sleep A = 1; P = 3	Sleep A = 1; P = 3
8–9 A.M.	↓	↓	↓
9–10 A.M.	↓	↓	↓
10–11 A.M.	↓	Get up A = 2; P = 1	↓
11 A.M.–12 P.M.	Get up A = 2; P = 1	Watch TV A = 1; P = 3	↓
12–1 P.M.	Eat lunch A = 1; P = 5	Eat lunch A = 1; P = 5	Get up A = 2; P = 1
1–2 P.M.	Take bus A = 3; P = 1	Watch TV A = 1; P = 2.5	Eat lunch A = 1; P = 7
2–3 P.M.	Go to appointment A = 7; P = 1	↓	Take care of neighbor's cat A = 4; P = 4
3–4 P.M.	Take bus A = 3; P = 1	↓	Paid bills A = 4; P = 1
4–5 P.M.	Watch TV A = 2; P = 4	Nap A = 1; P = 3	Watch TV A = 2; P = 4
5–6 P.M.	↓	↓	↓
6–7 P.M.	Eat dinner A = 2; P = 6	Eat dinner A = 2; P = 6	Eat dinner A = 2; P = 6
7–8 P.M.	Watch TV A = 2; P = 4	Bake brownies A = 2; P = 8	Go to the store A = 3; P = 3
8–9 P.M.	↓	Watch TV A = 1; P = 2.5	Eat ice cream A = 1; P = 9
9–10 P.M.	Eat snack A = 1; P = 8	↓	Watch TV A = 2; P = 4
10–11 P.M.	↓	Eat five brownies A = 1; P = 7	↓
11 P.M.–12 A.M.	Sleep A = 1; P = 3	Sleep A = 1; P = 3	Sleep A = 1; P = 3

FIGURE 8.4 Excerpt from Ellen's Activity Log.

addition to the processes of change relevant to all of the strategies to manage unpleasant emotions, the scheduling of pleasant, meaningful activities also utilizes contingency management, as group members get rewards from their environment that are different than the rewards they experienced by engaging in addictive behavior.

Controlled Breathing and Muscle Relaxation

In many instances, people become anxious when they perceive that they are in a situation that is uncontrollable or unpredictable. Many symptoms of anxiety are physical in nature (e.g., shallow breathing, muscle tension), and when they are experienced, anxious individuals often interpret them in a catastrophic manner (Clark, 1986). A vicious cycle ensues, such that increased anxiety makes these physical symptoms more noticeable, which in turn increases anxiety and the perception that one is out of control. Patients who are angry, in contrast, do not experience distress because of a perception of uncontrollability and unpredictability; rather, they focus on some perceived injustice (A. T. Beck, 1999). However, they often experience similar physical symptoms as do anxious patients. Controlled breathing and muscle relaxation strategies are particularly useful for managing these physical symptoms of anxiety and anger.

Controlled breathing allows patients who are anxious to regulate the amount of air that is going in and out of their body, which reinforces a sense of controllability over one physical symptom of anxiety and prevents their breathing disruption from culminating in hyperventilation (Craske & Barlow, 2008). Controlled breathing also regulates angry individuals' breathing, but with the goal of reducing the amount of affect they are experiencing so that they can use their problem-solving skills and think before acting on aggressive impulse. In both instances, controlled breathing also serves as a distraction strategy away from the high levels of anxiety and anger.

Below we describe one simple approach to controlled breathing:

- Teach group members about the difference between shallow breathing and diaphragmatic breathing. One is breathing shallowly if his or her shoulders move up and down with each breath. One is using diaphragmatic breathing if his or her stomach expands, like a balloon, on each in-breath and deflates with each out-breath. Have group members practice each type of breathing and ensure that they know what it feels like to engage in diaphragmatic breathing.
- Obtain a mood rating (e.g., degree of anxiety, anger, or other unpleasant mood state) before engaging in the controlled breathing exercise.

- Ask group members to close their eyes. If some group members express discomfort with closing their eyes, ask them to fix their gaze on one spot in the room.
- Guide group members in inhaling with their mouth or nose to a count of two and exhaling with their mouth or nose to a count of four, using diaphragmatic breathing. Continue this process for 10 consecutive breaths.
- Obtain another mood rating (e.g., degree of anxiety, anger, or other unpleasant mood state) after engaging in the controlled breathing exercise.
- Facilitate discussion among group members about the degree to which this strategy was helpful in reducing an aversive mood state. Encourage practice with the strategy.

This approach to controlled breathing is one of many that therapists incorporate into their clinical practice (Bourne, 2010; Reilly et al., 2002; Muñoz et al., 2000), and any one of them is appropriate to integrate into a CTAG if the facilitators decide that it would benefit the majority of the group members. The most important point for facilitators to keep in mind is that providing a rationale for the use of controlled breathing is crucial so that patients "buy into" it and make the commitment to practice on a regular basis.

Muscle relaxation works in a similar manner as controlled breathing, but it targets the physical symptoms of muscle tension, rather than shallow breathing. That is, it helps patients who are anxious to gain a sense of controllability and predictability over one physical symptom, and it helps patients who are angry to calm down before engaging in an aggressive response. Muscle relaxation also distracts patients from their unpleasant emotional experiences because it requires that they apply focused concentration to relaxing particular muscle groups. As we saw with controlled breathing, there are a number of protocols available (Bourne, 2010; Reilly et al., 2002; Velasquez et al., 2001; Muñoz et al., 2000), and the facilitator can choose the protocol with which he or she feels most comfortable. Group members may also download audio files from the Internet that may aid in their practice (e.g., *www.hws.edu/studentlife/media/CC%20Website%20Relax%20Steve.mp3*). Below is a simple protocol that we use in our CTAGs:

- Obtain a mood rating (e.g., degree of anxiety, anger, or other unpleasant mood state) before engaging in the muscle relaxation exercise.
- Invite group members to find a comfortable position in their seats, ensuring that they are not sitting rigidly.

- Dim the lights, and invite group members to close their eyes if they choose to do so.
- Consider beginning the exercise with a controlled breathing protocol, such as the one described previously.
- Guide group members as they tense each major muscle group for 10 seconds and release the tension for 20 seconds. Major muscle groups include feet, calves, quadriceps, buttocks, abdomen, groin, biceps, triceps, forearms, fists, neck, jaws, eyes, and forehead. Specific strategies for tensing muscle groups include clenching fists, curling arms as if doing a bicep curl, raising the shoulders toward the ears, and tensing muscles in the neck and face by making a face (Reilly et al., 2002).
- Obtain another mood rating (e.g., degree of anxiety, anger, or other unpleasant mood state) after engaging in the muscle relaxation exercise.
- Facilitate discussion among group members about the degree to which this strategy was helpful in reducing an aversive mood state. Encourage practice with the strategy.

IMPROVING PROBLEM-SOLVING SKILLS

Many patients with addictions report feeling overwhelmed as they try to put their lives back together during their recovery. Common problems they need to address include becoming employed, securing a favorable living arrangement, getting out of debt, and managing multiple appointments for medical, psychiatric, and social services. However, many of these patients lack the problem-solving skills necessary to address simultaneously these areas of their lives that are crucial for getting on the road to recovery. In fact, engaging in the addictive behavior often served as their solution for managing or escaping difficult life circumstances in the past. In this section, we describe five steps for effective problem solving: (1) identifying and prioritizing the problems, (2) brainstorming potential solutions, (3) evaluating potential solutions, (4) implementing a solution, and (5) evaluating the solution (Bieling et al., 2006; D'Zurilla & Nezu, 2007). These problem-solving steps achieve the self-liberation process of change, in that they help group members become aware of options for solving their problems and provide support in making better choices in their lives.

Identifying and Prioritizing Problems

Group members are often dealing with a large number of problems in their lives, which can be scary and overwhelming to them. We have witnessed many group members who simply shut down when they become over-whelmed, avoiding their problems and allowing their problems to build and build. The first step in problem solving, then, is often to clearly identify problems that need to be addressed and prioritize their importance. In most instances, the highest-priority problem will be the one that is addressed first, although at times, group members choose to first address a problem that is of lower priority but that is perceived as being more easily addressed than the others. Consider this vignette with Brian, when he reported being overwhelmed with his life problems:

BRIAN: I'm screwed. My wife could leave me at any minute. We're at risk of losing our home because I squandered our money. And now, work is slow, and I'm not bringing in enough. (*shaking head*) It's really all too much. I'm not sure how I will get out of this.

ELLEN: (*leans over and gives Brian's hand a squeeze*)

FACILITATOR 1: It strikes me that many of you have mentioned that you are overwhelmed with your problems. Might it be helpful to focus today's group on problem solving?

(*Group members nod their heads.*)

BRIAN: I could sure use it.

FACILITATOR 2: Those of you who have been in the group for some time and who have been part of previous discussions on problem solving, do you remember what the first step in solving a problem is?

BRIAN: (*laughing sarcastically*) I must have missed that discussion last time I attended these group sessions.

ELLEN: Isn't it just figuring out exactly what your problems are?

FACILITATOR 1: You're absolutely right. Identify the problem. And if there is more than one problem, prioritize their importance. (*turning to Brian*) I think I heard you mention three problems. What were those, again?

BRIAN: (*sighing and closing his eyes for a moment*) My wife, mort-gage payments, and no work. But that's just the tip of the iceberg. My tooth has been real sensitive, so I think I need dental work. And a light keeps coming on in my truck. I think it needs to go to the shop. (*pausing*) I've been putting off thinking about this because I don't want to know how much it will cost.

FACILITATOR 2: It sounds like things are really difficult for you right now. To summarize, it sounds like the problems on your plate right now are a strained relationship with your wife, being behind in mortgage payments, not enough work, a sore tooth, and your truck needing some repair. Am I right?

BRIAN: Yeah, that's it.

FACILITATOR 2: *(turning to the group)* When you all have faced many problems at once, how did you go about deciding which one to address first?

DAVE: That's the million dollar question. They all needed to be dealt with, like, yesterday.

MICHAEL: I guess you just have to prioritize them.

FACILITATOR 2: And how does one go about prioritizing?

ALLISON: Maybe rate it on a scale of 1–10? So the problem that gets a 10 can be the first one you start to solve.

BRIAN: But I would give a 10 to everything.

FACILITATOR 1: Allison's point is well taken. You can certainly rate each problem for its level of importance and first tackle the highest-rated problem. But, in instances like Brian's, when all of the problems are high priority, then other ways of prioritizing must be considered. For example, perhaps one problem is easier to solve than the others, and attending to it right away would build momentum and confidence to solve the other problems. Or, perhaps one problem can't be addressed until another one is solved.

BRIAN: I didn't think of that. I guess I can't find more work and make more money, or hell, even get myself to the dentist, if my truck isn't working. So maybe I should get that checked out first.

As they work with group members to prioritize their problems, facilitators can illustrate the prioritization process using the group itself as an example, as they have to prioritize group members' issues in order to determine the focus of each group session. In instances in which it is clear that group members are struggling to prioritize their problems, facilitators can guide them in gaining practice with systematically laying out each problem, its immediate and long-term consequences, and how detrimental each of those consequences would be. All of that information could be used to evaluate the importance of the problems to be addressed.

Brainstorming Potential Solutions

When patients are depressed or overwhelmed, they often fall into the trap of dismissing potential solutions to problems before objectively evaluating their merit. Thus, a crucial step in the problem-solving process is to brainstorm all possible solutions to problems, taking care not to judge them until the brainstorming process is complete. In our experience, solutions that, at first sound "off-the-wall" or difficult to implement, often inform a different and effective way of solving the problem that group members would have never considered, had they forgone the brainstorming process. Group members often find that brainstorming can be one of the most enjoyable activities in CTAGs, as they can be as creative as possible in generating potential solutions to one another's problems. The challenge for facilitators in guiding group members through the brainstorming process is to identify and address unhelpful cognitions that have the potential to thwart the open-minded generation of solutions (e.g., "I would never do this," "This will never work"). Our vignette continues after Brian decided to first address the potential repairs to his truck. Although a logical solution to the problem is to take the truck to a mechanic, Brian identified the more specific problem of needing to first identify a trustworthy mechanic:

> BRIAN: I don't even know where to start. My old mechanic retired and closed up his shop. I need to find a new mechanic, but I'm worried that they'll take me for everything I've got.
>
> FACILITATOR 1: So, how would you put words to the *specific* problem you're facing with the truck?
>
> BRIAN: I need to find a mechanic I can actually trust.
>
> FACILITATOR 2: This is a nice opportunity to practice the second step of problem solving, which is brainstorming. Who knows what brainstorming is?
>
> ALLISON: It's when you list all of the different ways of doing something, right?
>
> FACILITATOR 2: You got it, it's generating all possible solutions to a problem, without judging them or dismissing them, before deciding on a specific solution. Why might this be important?
>
> MICHAEL: Well, it's important to look at all your options before making a decision.
>
> ELLEN: Yes, sometimes it's easy to think you know how to solve a problem, when you really don't.
>
> FACILITATOR 2: Brian, can we brainstorm possible solutions with you?
>
> BRIAN: Yeah.
>
> FACILITATOR 2: (*gestures to the group to begin brainstorming*)

ELLEN: Maybe you could go on the Internet and read reviews of nearby mechanics?

BRIAN: Yeah, but I don't have time for that. I really need to focus on getting more work.

FACILITATOR 1: (*gently*) You're not obligated to do any of these solutions, Brian. Remember, right now we're just identifying all possibilities. I know it's very important for you to get more work. But, as we established a little while ago, it sounds like it's important to have your truck working in order to carry out any work that you get. Yes?

BRIAN: Yeah, I guess.

DAVE: I could tell you where to go. My buddy owns a shop.

FACILITATOR 2: Ah, yes. Recommendations from others.

MICHAEL: Could you go and get a few estimates? That way, you can compare prices and also get a feel for how the shop works before making a decision.

[The group members continue to brainstorm solutions, including choosing a mechanic from the yellow pages, going to the mechanic who is located closest to Brian's home, and choosing not to go to a mechanic and seeing whether the problem goes away. The group even began to have fun with one another and generate "off-the-wall" solutions, such as having Dave and his father repair the truck.]

Evaluating Potential Solutions

Once all potential solutions have been identified, the group can conduct an advantages–disadvantages analysis to evaluate each solution and weigh the pros and cons. Typical issues to consider in an advantages–disadvantages analysis include (1) cost, (2) time, (3) feasibility, (4) likelihood of success, (5) potential adverse consequences to implementing the solution, and (6) the degree to which the group member possesses the skills necessary to implement the solution. It is important for facilitators to be aware of unhelpful cognitions that might color the advantages–disadvantages analysis (e.g., overestimating the likelihood of failure of the solutions) and to use the cognitive strategies described in Chapter 7 to address them.

After evaluating the advantages and disadvantages of each potential solution, the facilitators guide group members in using that information to decide upon a specific solution. In many instances, the solutions are not mutually exclusive, and the group member might find that implementing two solutions, or a combination of the parts of two solutions, would be in his or her best interest. The end result is a well-thought-out solution that has taken into account short- and long-term consequences and feasibility. In Brian's case, he decided that he would spend the time to research reviews of mechanics on the Internet and seek out recommendations from others, as during the advantages–disadvantages analysis, it became clear that cost is the most important issue to keep in mind. Had he dismissed these solutions during the brainstorming process, as was his first inclination, he might have chosen a solution that would take less of his time but that would have, potentially, resulted in a higher cost of services.

Implementing a Solution

In order to increase the likelihood that group members will actually implement the solution they identify, facilitators ensure that they can articulate the specific manner in which they will implement the solution, that they have the resources to implement the solution, and that they identify any obstacles that might interfere with implementing solutions and to plan, in advance, ways to overcome those obstacles. In many instances, it is helpful for group members to use imagery rehearsal to imagine themselves successfully implementing the solution. It is also helpful for group members to commit to a time frame in which they will implement the solution so that they are not deterred by avoidance, procrastination, or forgetfulness. The following vignette illustrates the manner in which these aims were accomplished with Brian:

> FACILITATOR 1: So, after all of this discussion, Brian, you have decided to do some research on the Internet and get recommendations from others to choose a mechanic.
>
> BRIAN: (*nods and smiles*)
>
> FACILITATOR 1: Tell us how, specifically, you will do this.
>
> BRIAN: First, I'm going to ask my neighbor for a recommendation, since he just had some work done on his car. And, I already have Dave's suggestion as well. Then, I'll look up reviews on those two mechanics on the Internet, and I'll also keep my eyes peeled to see if there are good reviews of any other mechanic.
>
> FACILITATOR 2: And what will you do with this information?
>
> BRIAN: I'll just choose the one with the best reviews, especially if the reviews say the guy is trustworthy or inexpensive.
>
> FACILITATOR 1: Terrific. And when will you do this?
>
> BRIAN: I'll do it when I get home. I don't have to work for the rest of the day.

FACILITATOR 2: Can you think of anything that might get in the way of implementing this solution?

BRIAN: (*pausing, thinking*) Well, I've been putting this off because I really don't want to find out that my truck is on its last legs. I guess if I start thinking about that, I might chicken out.

ELLEN: You won't chicken out, Brian. You worked hard on this in session.

FACILITATOR 2: I agree, Brian. You have worked hard. In the event that you start to feel anxious and feel yourself moving toward avoidance of doing this, what can you do?

BRIAN: I need to tell myself that the avoidance won't get me anywhere. (*looking at the group slyly*) Heck, maybe I'll do yet another advantages–disadvantages analysis of calling a mechanic or waiting. (*Group chuckles.*)

If facilitators sense that a group member is ambivalent about implementing a solution, they can ask the group member the likelihood of following through on a scale of 0–10 (0 = *not at all likely*, 10 = *very likely*). If the group member responds with a number less than nine, then the group can work further using the cognitive behavioral strategies described in this chapter and in Chapter 7 to identify the source of ambivalence and increase motivation.

Evaluating the Solution

After group members have decided upon solutions to their specific problems, a logical homework assignment is for them to implement those solutions. When they return to the next group session, facilitators can take the opportunity to implement the final step of problem-solving training—evaluation of the solution. Factors to consider in the evaluation of the solution include (1) to what degree did the solution achieve the desired outcome? (2) what were the obstacles encountered in implementing the solution? and (3) what did the group members learn from this exercise that they can apply to other problems in their lives? Facilitators are encouraged to set up the discussion of solution evaluation from a "win–win" perspective—the solution either achieved the desired outcome, or if it did not, the implementation of the proposed solution yielded valuable information that can help the group member hone his or her skill in problem solving. In addition, facilitators can used the cognitive strategies described in Chapter 7 to address any unhelpful statements expressed by group members during the evaluation process (e.g., "It didn't work, so I'm a loser"). Consider the evaluation process with Brian in this vignette:

DAVE: Well, what happened? Did you find out what was wrong with your truck?

BRIAN: (*smiling sheepishly*) Yes, I did. (*turning to the group*) Would you believe there was nothing wrong with it? The check engine light just came on because I needed an oil change.

ELLEN: That's incredible. What good luck you had!

FACILITATOR 2: Let's hear a bit about how you implemented the problem-solving work we did last week. You had decided upon a strategy to find a trustworthy mechanic.

BRIAN: I did what we talked about. I talked to my neighbor when I got home from group, and I got on the Internet and read some reviews. It didn't take me as long as I thought. The reviews made it pretty clear which mechanics are good, you know, well respected, and which ones aren't.

ALLISON: Where did you end up going?

BRIAN: To the one who fixed my neighbor's car. It's less than a mile away from my place. And the guy got four out of five stars on his reviews.

FACILITATOR 1: Did you encounter any obstacles in your search for a mechanic?

BRIAN: Not really. But when I got home, I started to feel really nervous about it. The "What ifs?" jumped in my head again. I didn't think I could take it if the truck needed thousands of dollars in repairs.

FACILITATOR 2: What did you learn from this experience?

BRIAN: (*sighing*) I guess that there's no point in avoiding my problems. They aren't going to go away. And I could have created my own damage if I would have waited much longer, since the oil really needed to be changed.

FACILITATOR 2: Last week, you were overwhelmed with a number of problems. Now that you have addressed this one, how are you feeling about the others?

BRIAN: My problems seem never ending. But it was nice to get rid of a worry. And since I knew my truck is OK, I've actually been looking more actively for other jobs, and I think one is going to work out.

ELLEN: That's wonderful, Brian!

LEADING A HEALTHY LIFESTYLE

Although no one necessarily likes to deal with problems and setbacks in life, it is much easier to handle them in the context of a healthy, balanced lifestyle. Many patients who have struggled with addictions led chaotic lives, and they might not know what is meant by leading a healthy lifestyle. Facilitators can provide psychoeducation to group members about the importance of making healthy lifestyle choices, such as eating regular and nutritious meals, keeping a regular sleep schedule, and adhering to medical and mental health treatment programs. In order to achieve these aims, facilitators often use many of the strategies described in this volume so far, such as problem solving and behavioral experiments. Sometimes patients are unconvinced that making lifestyle changes can have a substantial impact on their mood, ability to handle stress, and manage their urges and cravings. In these cases, it can be helpful for group members to monitor their diet, sleep, and mood in between sessions so that they can see firsthand the manner in which lifestyle and symptoms are associated. Psychoeducation and monitoring of these issues work through the consciousness raising process of change, and lifestyle changes are achieved by counterconditioning.

In a recent CTAG session, Facilitator 1 noted that Dave seemed particularly tired and irritable. When he asked Dave if he was OK, he learned that Dave stayed up most of the night watching television and had to be at work by 8:00 A.M. The following is a vignette in which the facilitators use a cognitive behavioral approach to educating Dave and the rest of the group about maintaining a healthy lifestyle and prompt group members to make positive changes in their lifestyles:

FACILITATOR 1: I'm curious about whether you notice a relation between the amount of sleep you get and your mood the following day.

DAVE: (*exasperated*) I'm fine. I never get that much sleep, so this is no different.

FACILITATOR 1: What about the rest of you? Do any of you notice a relation between your sleep and mood?

ALLISON: I sure do. If I don't get 8 hours of sleep per night, then I'm a grouch.

MICHAEL: When I don't get enough sleep, I feel really groggy at work, and I know I'm not handling my clients the way I should be. I make a lot of mistakes.

DAVE: Yeah, well, I can do my job with my eyes closed, so none of this applies to me.

FACILITATOR 1: Let's take a step back for a moment. Dave's position is that sleep does not affect his mood and functioning. But Allison and Michael are indicating that there *is* a relation between sleep, mood, and functioning. Dave, would you be willing to do a test of these ideas in the next week?

DAVE: (*puzzled look on his face*)

FACILITATOR 1: Kind of like what you did when you predicted that your girlfriend was pregnant—you went out and got the pregnancy test to gather additional information before you concluded that she was pregnant.

DAVE: (*sarcastically*) So you want me to take a test to see if I need to sleep better?

FACILITATOR 1: Well, not a test that you can buy in a store. But you can make up the test on your own. Do you have a calendar?

DAVE: Yeah, hanging on my refrigerator.

FACILITATOR 1: Would you be willing to jot down two pieces of information on your calendar each day—the number of hours you slept the previous night, and your mood on a 0–100 scale? (*Facilitator 1 does not ask Dave to make any additional ratings, such as his level of functioning or intensity of cravings, because Dave is giving signals that he is not entirely invested in this intervention.*)

DAVE: And the purpose of this is what?

FACILITATOR 1: I'm glad you asked. The purpose is to see whether there is any association between your sleep and the quality of your mood the next day. If your mood stays the same no matter how many hours you slept the previous night, then you're accurate in your assessment that your sleep does not affect your mood. But if you do see an association, then you might be more motivated to make an adjustment to your sleep schedule.

DAVE: (*yawning*) I guess I can do that.

The facilitators went on to ask other group members if there are any other lifestyle factors associated with their mood, ability to function, and/or urges and cravings, and they helped them to devise similar experiments. The following vignette occurred at the subsequent session, when the facilitators asked group members to discuss their homework assignments:

FACILITATOR 1: OK, Dave, what's the verdict?

DAVE: (*begrudgingly*) OK, OK. The group was right. I was a hell of lot less irritable when I actually got a good night's sleep.

FACILITATOR 2: It takes a lot of courage to face the group and tell them that your experiment told you something other than what you expected. So what are you going to do with this information?

DAVE: I guess I'll try to sleep more. But, I don't know, I'm not that optimistic that things will change. Whenever I try to go to bed at a decent hour, I can't fall asleep.

[The facilitators proceed to assess the circumstances surrounding Dave's sleep schedule, educate the group about healthy sleep habits, and use problem solving to identify ways each group member could implement changes into his or her sleep schedule.]

SUMMARY

The development of coping skills involves the application of cognitive and behavioral strategies to manage cravings and urges, repair existing relationships, develop healthy new relationships, manage unpleasant emotions, improve problem-solving abilities, and make healthy lifestyle changes. Many of these coping skills are geared toward reducing cravings and urges and rebuilding group members' lives in the aftermath of their destructive behavior. However, it is also permissible for facilitators to address coping skills that will be helpful in managing life's problems more generally, even if they seem unrelated to group members' history of addictions, because such life problems make individuals vulnerable to a slip or relapse. The goal of a focus on coping skills is to help group members develop a wide range of strategies that can be applied to future stress and adversity so that they can cope without resorting to addictive behavior.

FORM 8.1. Activity Log

	Day 1	Day 2	Day 3	Day 4	Day 5	Day 6	Day 7
12–1 A.M.							
1–2 A.M.							
2–3 A.M.							
3–4 A.M.							
4–5 A.M.							
5–6 A.M.							
6–7 A.M.							
7–8 A.M.							
8–9 A.M.							
9–10 A.M.							
10–11 A.M.							

(cont.)

Activity Log *(page 2 of 2)*

	Day 1	Day 2	Day 3	Day 4	Day 5	Day 6	Day 7
11 A.M.–12 P.M.							
12–1 P.M.							
1–2 P.M.							
2–3 P.M.							
3–4 P.M.							
4–5 P.M.							
5–6 P.M.							
6–7 P.M.							
7–8 P.M.							
8–9 P.M.							
9–10 P.M.							
10–11 P.M.							
11 P.M.–12 A.M.							

CHAPTER 9 | Homework and Closure

Two components of the CTAG promote consolidation of learning: (1) the homework assignment, and (2) closure that occurs at the end of the session. *Homework* refers to between-session work that group members complete so that they can begin to implement the cognitive and behavioral strategies in their daily lives. Completion of homework gives group members valuable information about ways to manage urges, cravings, unpleasant mood states, and/or the consequences of their addictive behavior, which they can later share with their fellow group members in order to receive feedback and further hone their coping abilities. *Closure* refers to the process of concluding or ending the group in a constructive, positive, effective manner for all group members. Strategies for developing effective homework assignments and for effectively closing group sessions are considered in this chapter.

HOMEWORK

Homework is regarded as an essential component of every cognitive therapy protocol. There is evidence that a higher level of compliance with homework is associated with greater gains in individual therapy (Addis & Jacobson, 2000), and there is no reason to believe that this same association would not hold true for people who participate in group therapy. Homework assignments allow group members to practice the cognitive and behavioral strategies considered in group sessions in their own environment, outside of the session. Many group members make negative predictions about their ability to achieve goals (e.g., "I'll never be hired for a job with my history"), and homework assignments allow them to test out these predictions. Thus, homework assignments help group members to see, from an experiential perspective, the manner in which the contents of the group sessions apply to their lives so that they can begin to make positive changes and healthy decisions.

Development of Homework Assignments

Although we discuss the development of homework assignments in this final clinical chapter, in reality, homework assignments can be developed at any point in the session that is relevant. In fact, we encourage facilitators *not* to wait until the last few minutes of a session to develop a homework assignment, as there likely will not be sufficient time to develop a compelling activity that will resonate with group members. We find that the development of a homework assignment is most effective when it flows naturally from group discussion in session.

Figure 9.1 summarizes characteristics of effective cognitive therapy homework assignments. Collaboration between the therapist and the patient is a key tenet of cognitive therapy, and that principle is especially important to keep in mind as homework assignments are developed. If group members perceive that homework is being "assigned" to them by the facilitators, or if facilitators have to "convince" group members to do the assignment, the likelihood of follow-through is lowered. Thus, it is important that

---

- Ensure that group members understand and are on board with the rationale for the homework assignment.
- Develop homework assignment collaboratively, such that each group member tailors the assignment to his or her unique needs and learning style while accomplishing the same overall goal.
- Include one straightforward activity in the homework assignment.
- Ensure that the homework assignment logically follows the activity that was the focus of the session.
- Start the homework assignment in session.
- Encourage group members to write down the assignment on a piece of paper or in their smartphones.
- Have group members rate the likelihood of homework completion on a 0–10 scale (0 = *not likely*, 10 = *very likely*), and address instances in which ratings are less than a 9.
- Ensure that the homework assignment represents a "win-win" situation, so that problems with homework completion are viewed as providing useful information.

FIGURE 9.1. Strategies to improve homework compliance.

group members actively contribute to the development of the homework assignment in order to ensure that (1) they understand the rationale for the homework assignment and the specific manner it is expected to make a difference in their lives, and (2) the assignment is customized to their unique needs and learning style. Group members who are convinced that the homework assignment is meaningful to their lives and that they have the ability to complete the assignment are most likely to actually do it in the time in between sessions.

Consider the vignette we presented on pages 134 to 137 of Chapter 7, in which the group agreed to extend the exercise that they had completed in session and monitor their thoughts in between sessions. When Dave expressed skepticism about the exercise by stating he did not know whether he would complete the assignment and by asking "What's the point?" the facilitators enlisted other group members to explain their understanding of the rationale for the assignment. In addition, the facilitators created a collaborative environment such that each group member considered a way to tailor the assignment to his or her unique needs and learning style while still accomplishing the same goal.

Facilitators are also cognizant of many other factors that contribute to the development of an effective homework assignment. In the vignette in Chapter 7, the homework assignment consisted of one straightforward activity—the monitoring of thoughts. In our experience, developing an especially complex homework assignment, or assigning more than one activity, decreases the likelihood of completion. This is so because some group members get overwhelmed when they perceive there is too much to keep track of in between sessions, whereas some other group members become confused and leave the session not fully understanding what the between-session work involves. In addition, the homework assignment described in Chapter 7 logically followed the activity that was the focus of the session; thus, in essence, it was started in session. Starting the homework assignment in session increases the likelihood of success because group members have a model to follow when they attempt it outside of session, and they have already shown themselves that they have the capacity to complete it (thereby increasing self-efficacy).

The likelihood of homework completion also increases when group members write down the assignment. In this vignette, each person left the group with a Thought Record, with the instructions clearly written on the sheet. In other instances, group members can simply write down the skill they will practice or activity to which they will commit to doing. Form 9.1 (at the end of the chapter) is an example of a simple template on which group members can write down their homework assignment. Notice that this sheet provides space for group members to record the frequency with which they plan on doing the assignment and the times that they anticipate doing this. Recording this information often enhances their commitment and likelihood of follow-through. The space for group members to write what they learned from the assignment is another opportunity for group members to consolidate their learning so that they will be able to use the CTAG principle at other times in their lives, even when it is not assigned for homework.

It is important that facilitators do not make the assumption that group members are sure to complete the homework assignment. Thus, once the homework assignment is developed and agreed upon by group members and facilitators, facilitators ask each group member for the likelihood that he or she will complete the assignment on a scale of 0–10 (0 = *very unlikely*, 10 = *very likely*). If group members indicate a likelihood of less than 9, then it is important for facilitators to help group members identify obstacles that they expect to encounter in completing the assignment. A problem-solving approach, as described in Chapter 8, can be useful in addressing these obstacles and developing ways to overcome them. After consideration of potential obstacles, if group members continue to provide estimates that are lower than a 9 on the 10-point scale, then facilitators can revisit the assignment in order to make it more manageable. Consider the continuation of this vignette, when the facilitators were surprised to learn that Michael had doubts about completing the assignment:

FACILITATOR 1: On a scale of 0–10, with 0 being very unlikely, and 10 being very likely, how likely is it that each of you will complete this Thought Record in between now and the next time we see you?

ALLISON: Oh, definitely a 10. I'm really getting a lot out of this.

ELLEN: Me too, 10.

BRIAN: You know me, I'm kind of hit and miss with homework. But I'm starting to pull things together, and I've done my homework the past couple of weeks. So I'll give it a 9.

DAVE: I'm with Brian, a 9.

MICHAEL: I think it's worthwhile, but I'm going out of town on business, so I'm not sure if I'll be able to get to this.

FACILITATOR 2: (*gently*) Michael, if I remember correctly, the last time you went out of town on business was the last time you slipped, is that right?

MICHAEL: (*sheepishly*) Yeah, that's right. Except this time will be a lot different because I've stayed away from the stuff for over 6 months.

ELLEN: You've made so much progress in group and have shown yourself and us that you can deal with your urges and cravings. But

I'm wondering if this is actually the *perfect* time to complete a Thought Record because this a high-risk situation.

MICHAEL: Yeah, I know. But I'll be in meetings all day, and then I'll go out to dinner. I don't want to complete a Thought Record in front of all of my colleagues!

(*Group chuckles.*)

FACILITATOR 1: Do you agree, in theory, that the Thought Record would be helpful for you to identify urges that come up while you're out of town?

MICHAEL: In theory, yes, I've used it before, and it's helped me to remember that the urge is something I experience in the short term, and I have long-term goals to worry about, like rebuilding my wife's trust in me.

FACILITATOR 1: OK, let's brainstorm opportunities to complete the Thought Record while you're out of town. (*involves the group in identifying creative places and times to complete the exercise*)

MICHAEL: OK, you all have given me some good ideas. I guess you're right, people type things in their BlackBerries all the time during meetings, and no one has to know what they're writing. (*pausing*) Yeah, this is really good. I think I was getting too confident, you know, thinking that I have mastered all of this. I think doing this will be a nice check and balance for me.

A central feature of homework assignments is that they should be readily achievable. It is helpful for facilitators to guide group members in developing assignments that represent a "win–win" situation, much as we saw in Chapter 7 regarding the development of behavioral experiments. If group members successfully complete the homework assignment, then, presumably, they have acquired a skill; practiced or honed a skill; refuted a negative thought, prediction, or belief; or obtained an important insight about the interplay of cognition, emotion, and addictive behavior. However, facilitators also encounter instances when group members do not successfully complete their homework assignment, either because the group members did not attempt the assignment, or because the group members attempted it but were unable to carry it out. Facilitators can anticipate these outcomes in advance and assure group members that, if the homework does not work out, it nevertheless provides important information. For example, it might let the facilitators know that they need to take more time to articulate the rationale for the practice of cognitive and behavioral strategies, or that the group needs more in-session practice with the strategies. It also might point to the fact that group members experience unhelpful cognitions about doing the homework (e.g., "I'm a loser, so things will never change") that must be addressed and evaluated in session so that group members can have a more helpful cognitive stance as they attempt future homework assignments. Facilitators communicate to group members their confidence in their belief that the homework assignment will be helpful for members in their recovery, but they also take care to let group members know that they are welcome back if they do not complete their assignment in order to further brainstorm ways to customize the treatment for them.

The example presented in the chapter to this point illustrates an instance in which all group members agree to complete the same homework assignment, albeit with some modifications to meet the needs of individual group members. In other instances, group members agree to a homework assignment that reflects one theme (e.g., repairing relationships with close others, managing urges and cravings), but each group member identifies a specific skill to practice in between sessions. Each group member, then, might be practicing a different skill or activity, but each skill or activity helps him or her to achieve the goal that was the topic of the group session. For example, during a session that was devoted to coping skills to manage urges and cravings, for homework, Michael agreed to use imagery to imagine his wife's face if he were caught with another woman when he experienced sexual urges, Allison agreed to call a friend when she experienced urges to smoke, Brian agreed to complete an advantages–disadvantages analysis when he experienced urges to gamble, Ellen agreed to imagine herself 50 pounds thinner and to work on the quilt for her niece's baby when she experienced urges to overeat, and Dave agreed to either work on his truck or go to a different friend's house to work on the friend's motorcycle when he experienced urges to drink or use drugs.

Whenever possible, it is important for group members to record the use of their coping skills so that they can track its application and effectiveness. Thus, the facilitators also encouraged group members to record the intensity of their urges and cravings (0 = *none*, 10 = *extreme*) before using the coping skill and after using the coping skill (see Form 9.2 at the end of the chapter). Not only does this intervention provide an opportunity for group members to record instances in which they used the coping skill, which increases accountability, but it also provides tangible evidence that speaks to the effectiveness of the coping skill. When group members see that the intensity of their urges and cravings decreases by implementing a particular coping skill, it increases the likelihood that they will use that skill in the future. The same pre–post recording approach can be used by group members to evaluate the effectiveness of skills in managing mood, relationships, and unhealthy lifestyle choices.

Although it is preferable that homework assignments be relatively similar for every group member to ensure consistency, on occasion, it is clear that a group member is struggling with a particular issue and that it would be in his or her best interest to focus on resolving that issue in the time in between sessions. In the next vignette, it became clear that Ellen's depression had worsened and that it was interfering with her commitment to implementing cognitive and behavioral strategies to manage her overeating addiction. The other group members in this session agreed to a homework assignment in which they would initiate contact with one family member or friend from whom they became estranged because of their addiction. However, because Ellen's clinical presentation was concerning to the facilitators, they obtained her commitment to take action to address her depressive symptoms. The following vignette took place during the time in which group members were identifying the person with whom they would initiate contact:

> FACILITATOR 1: Ellen, I have to admit that I'm a bit concerned about you today. You look tired, and you haven't said much in today's group. Does the homework the group is developing seem relevant to you at this moment?
>
> ELLEN: (*beginning to cry*) No, things are just awful right now! I haven't lost any weight, and I just sit around my apartment doing absolutely nothing. No one wants to hear from me. What kind of a life is this?
>
> ALLISON: (*reaches over and gives Ellen's hand a squeeze*)
>
> FACILITATOR 1: (*gently*) It seems to me that your depression has gotten a lot worse lately. Has it helped to use any of the skills that we discuss in group?
>
> ELLEN: What's the use? Things won't change. I don't have the energy to use the skills anyway.
>
> FACILITATOR 2: Does your psychiatrist know that you're feeling this badly?
>
> ELLEN: No, I only see her once every 3 months for a medication check. And even then, it's only for 20 minutes.
>
> FACILITATOR 1: When's your next appointment?
>
> ELLEN: (*choking on tears*) Not for a month and a half.
>
> FACILITATOR 1: I'm wondering if it should be a priority to get in contact with your psychiatrist and have a visit with her as soon as you can. Does this sound like something you can accomplish between now and our next group?
>
> ELLEN: I don't know. Probably not. It takes forever to speak with someone other than the switchboard. And even if I get in touch with a receptionist, she's usually booked for at least a few weeks.

FACILITATOR 1: Would you be willing to start this homework with me after group? Perhaps we can go to my office, and we can make the call together.

ELLEN: Well ... OK.

In this case, the facilitators chose not to address Ellen's multiple cognitive distortions for several reasons. First, the group was nearing the end its 90-minute session, and a focus exclusively on Ellen's problems would have prevented the remainder of the group members from committing to homework and gaining closure. Second, as mentioned in Chapter 5, facilitators are aware of group members' psychiatric history, and in this case, the facilitators knew that Ellen has been admitted to the hospital as an inpatient on two occasions for persistent suicidal ideation. Thus, they judged that it would be in her best interest to take immediate action in addressing her depressive symptoms. Facilitator 1 made the suggestion to work together with Ellen to call her psychiatrist because her response and tone of voice suggested that she would not follow through with making the call on her own. Moreover, he wanted to meet with her one-on-one to more thoroughly assess the extent of her depression and assess for suicidal thoughts and wishes. Not only were the facilitators successful in helping Ellen get an appointment for the subsequent afternoon, they also completed a safety plan with her (cf. Wenzel, Brown, & Beck, 2009) to ensure that there were concrete steps she could take in the event that she was feeling suicidal. This example illustrates the fact that the CTAG should not be the *only* form of treatment for group members who are experiencing comorbid psychiatric symptoms, as often these symptoms require more time and individualized attention.

Figure 9.2 lists some typical homework assignments that patients often complete in cognitive therapy, all of which can be done in the context of the CTAG. This list is far from exhaustive, and in reality, the only factor that limits that type of homework assignment designed is the imagination of the facilitators and group members. As has been seen in many instances in this volume, homework assignments might involve practicing some of the cognitive and behavioral strategies discussed in session. They also often involve using problem-solving skills to work toward reaching a goal such as preparing and submitting an application for a job. In some instances, there is an interpersonal component to homework assignments. Group members are encouraged to initiate, enhance, or repair a relationship with another individual by applying effective communication skills or engaging in a shared activity. Many of these assignments can also be used to disconfirm group members' beliefs that they are ineffective, that their situation will not change, and/or that others will be unresponsive to them.

- Implement a coping skill to manage urges and cravings.
- Complete a Four-Column or a Six-Column Thought Record.
- Develop or regularly consult a coping card.
- Engage in a pleasurable activity.
- Complete an activity monitoring or activity scheduling form.
- Practice controlled breathing at designated times.
- Practice muscle relaxation at designated times.
- Call a family member or friend.
- Use communication skills to negotiate a conflict.
- Attend or participate in an activity in which one might meet new people.
- Conduct a behavioral experiment designed in session.
- Conduct an advantages–disadvantages analysis.
- Implement the solution to a problem considered in session.
- Monitor a healthy living skill (e.g., sleep, meals) and its association with mood and/or urges and cravings.
- Implement one healthy living skill.

FIGURE 9.2. Typical homework assignments.

Review of the Previous Session's Homework

Because homework is given great emphasis in cognitive therapy, it is essential that facilitators review homework in the subsequent group session. Review of homework helps to weave a coherent thread across sessions. Some facilitators even have group members turn in written homework before the session starts so that they can review it and address successes and problems that may have arisen (Bieling et al., 2006). When facilitators neglect to review homework, they implicitly communicate the message that homework is not important or that group members are not accountable. Individuals who struggle with addictive behaviors, in particular, often have trouble with taking responsibility and accountability, so it is especially important in CTAGs to address the homework that had been assigned in the previous session.

Facilitators can use their clinical judgment in determining the most appropriate time to review homework with group members. This might occur in the introductions, especially in instances in which the group is small in number and composed of members who had attended the previous session and were privy to the homework assignment. In other instances, the session will continue to focus on the same or a related theme as it did in the previous week, and homework can be reviewed before additional cognitive and behavioral coping strategies are discussed. In fact, the successes and failures in completing homework assignments might determine, in part, the particular strategies that are focused on in the subsequent session. Thus, homework can be discussed as a logical lead in to discussion that will be continued from the previous week's session. In instances in which it is clear that the focus or theme of the group will be different than in the previous week, facilitators take time to review the previous week's homework before delving into the new topic.

When new members are present, or when returning group members are present who had not attended the previous week's session, facilitators are mindful to explain the previous homework assignment and obtain feedback about the manner in which the assignment has the potential to be relevant to their own recovery. The following vignette illustrates the review of the thought-monitoring homework assignment, taking care to incorporate the new group member introduced in Chapter 6, Rachel, into the discussion. Because the facilitators noted that there was a new member and also expected to continue to practice and add to cognitive restructuring skills in this session, they opted to review the homework after introductions and review of the cognitive model of addictions but before introducing skills for evaluating situational cognitions.

> FACILITATOR 1: One constant in every CTAG session is that group members commit to a homework assignment, so that they can practice the skills discussed in group in between sessions. And it just so happens that the homework from last week applies directly to the cognitive model of addiction that we just reviewed. Would anyone be willing to share what that homework assignment was and how it relates to the cognitive model?
>
> ELLEN: Well, what we are thinking or saying to ourselves has a large impact on our addictions, and even on how we feel. So our task was to jot down some of these thoughts that get us into trouble when we noticed them.
>
> FACILITATOR 1: Perhaps we can check in with the folks who were here last week to give them some feedback on their homework, and then, before introducing new skills, we can take a moment to consider how this exercise would apply to our new member, Rachel. Does that sound like a plan to everyone?
>
> (*Group members nod their heads.*)
>
> FACILITATOR 1: Who would like to start?
>
> MICHAEL: I can go. (*pausing*) It was a good thing that we talked about this in here last week before I went on my business trip because

I was really tempted. It was the first time away from the family in quite awhile. I found myself about to go right back to my old ways.

BRIAN: But you didn't?

MICHAEL: No, I didn't.

(*Group gives a sigh of relief.*)

MICHAEL: But it was really tough, much tougher than I had expected it to be.

FACILITATOR 2: What were some of the thoughts you recorded in your BlackBerry?

MICHAEL: I started going down the road of the facilitating thoughts. You know, things like "No one will ever know," or "I've been so good, I deserve just one slip."

FACILITATOR 2: Did those facilitating thoughts enhance your urges and cravings or minimize them?

MICHAEL: Oh, I can definitely see how they just made them worse. I came so close to actually doing it.

ELLEN: How did you stop yourself, Michael?

MICHAEL: Through a combination of things we've talked about in group. I did use that technique to imagine my wife's face if she found out. But I also reminded myself of how far I have come and that never, not ever, have there been positive long-term consequences to having a fling with a random person.

FACILITATOR 1: Thank you, Michael, for candidly sharing the thoughts you experienced and powerfully they were related to your urges and cravings. You've also anticipated what we'll be working on in today's session—ways to construct alternative statements that you can say to yourselves in these instances in order to manage urges and cravings. Who else would like to share?

ALLISON: I can go. I found that my thoughts were mainly angry ones directed toward my husband and my mother-in-law, rather than ones about smoking. In fact, I actually had a pretty good week with the urges and cravings.

(*Some group members give a thumbs up.*)

ALLISON: But my husband and mother-in-law, they really got me down.

FACILITATOR 2: It sounds like you had two prominent emotional experiences this week—feeling angry and feeling down. What were the thoughts associated with those?

ALLISON: It was kind of the same thought over and over. Just that they don't care about me.

FACILITATOR 2: That statement, "They don't care about me," is a powerful thought that would likely be associated with feelings of anger and sadness in a lot of people, Allison.

(*Facilitators go on to check in with the other group members with their homework assignments.*)

FACILITATOR 1: Let's make sure we keep Rachel in the loop regarding this exercise. Rachel, we've heard a number of group members identify a link between thoughts running through their minds and urges, cravings, and unpleasant moods. How do you think this applies to you?

RACHEL: I think it will take me some time to catch on.

FACILITATOR 1: Do you buy the idea that our thoughts, moods, and behaviors like urges and cravings are interconnected?

RACHEL: Yeah, after listening to everyone, I think I do.

FACILITATOR 1: In today's session, we'll continue to focus on our thoughts and ways to respond to them adaptively. We often practice such exercises in pairs. So we'll be sure to pair you with someone who's been in the group for a while so that they can show you the ropes.

ELLEN: I'd be happy to work with you, Rachel.

RACHEL: (*looking relieved*) Thanks, that would be helpful.

This vignette illustrates two points. First, not only is it important to review each group member's homework, but it is also important to link their work back to the cognitive model so that the association among cognitions, moods, and behaviors is continually reinforced. Second, it is important for facilitators to strike a balance between including new group members (or group members who did not attend the previous week's session) into the discussion while not spending so much time with them that the need to "catch them up" assumes importance over the momentum built by the group members who completed their homework assignment. Pairing up new group members with seasoned group members is one approach for modeling CTAG structure, process, and strategy to people who did not attend the previous session. If feasible, facilitators can also invite these group members to stay after group in order to provide some individual instruction.

CTAG facilitators will undoubtedly encounter many instances in which group members do not complete the homework assignment. When this occurs, it is important for facilitators to address noncompliance in group; failure to do so inadvertently models that homework is not important. However, it is equally important to ensure that facilitators do not shame or reprimand group members for not completing the assignment. Instead, facilitators adopt a collaborative and constructive approach to ensure that group members are committed to the goals of the group. As stated earlier in this chapter, failure to complete a homework assignment can be regarded as important information that can be used to identify a skills deficit, interfering cognitions that can be addressed in the group session, or a need to individualize assignments even further. It also offers an opportunity to reeducate the group about the importance of homework and the rationale for the cognitive and behavioral strategies that are practiced during and between group sessions. The following vignette illustrates the manner in which the facilitators addressed homework noncompliance by two group members, Brian and Dave:

FACILITATOR 1: Before we move on to working further with our situational cognitions, I'd like to check in with Brian and Dave and determine what obstacles they encountered in completing the homework.

DAVE: Just didn't think of it, that's all.

BRIAN: I won't lie to you—this week has been awful. I just didn't have it in me to do it.

FACILITATOR 1: In my experience, forgetting to do the homework and not feeling like doing it are two common reasons why people often let the homework go. (*turning to the group*) Has anyone else ever experienced the obstacles?

MICHAEL: I did, early on. It just seemed like I was too busy to squeeze it in. So I either forgot about it altogether or put it off.

ELLEN: I've been in the same place as you're in, Brian, when things have seemed so bad that there was no point in doing the homework.

ALLISON: It took me a little bit to get used to doing the homework when I first started. But now that I come to group every week, it's just part of my routine.

FACILITATOR 1: Ah, so one way to overcome these obstacles is to make completion of your homework routine, so that it fits into your schedule.

MICHAEL: Yeah. And when you think about it, we're all spending a lot of time and energy coming to this group. So why wouldn't we want to do the homework so that we make sure our time is spent wisely?

FACILITATOR 2: Dave and Brian, what do both of you see as the point of homework?

BRIAN: I know I need to practice this stuff in order to get over my gambling addiction once and for all.

FACILITATOR 2: Yes, practicing the skills in between session. The next time you have a bad week, and you don't feel like doing your homework, what can you do to overcome that inertia?

BRIAN: I like what Michael said, to remember that it's up to me to make the most of this treatment. I guess I also have to remember that every time I quit coming to group, I had a lapse.

FACILITATOR 2: Good, Brian. It sounds like you've developed an alternative way of viewing the homework. Dave, what about you?

DAVE: I just really hate to write. And recording it in the phone still seems like writing.

FACILITATOR 1: Do you believe in the basic model, that addressing problematic thoughts and behaviors is central in overcoming addiction?

DAVE: Yeah, I guess, I don't know. But it just seems too much like school to me.

FACILITATOR 1: Tell you what, maybe the two of us can touch base after group and see if we can continue to put our heads together and figure out a way to tailor this to your unique needs and learning style.

DAVE: OK.

This vignette illustrates several common approaches to dealing with homework noncompliance. First, the facilitators initiated a discussion among the group as a whole to identify obstacles commonly experienced in completing homework. This discussion had the potential to illustrate to Brian and Dave that most, if not all, group members have experienced this from time to time, which reinforces a sense of universality. Moreover, it allowed group members to share insights regarding ways to overcome those obstacles. If needed, facilitators can take this discussion even further, such as by having group members generate very concrete ways to remember to do their homework (e.g., a Post-it Note on the medicine cabinet) and motivate themselves to do it (e.g., a coping card that lists the benefits of doing homework). Second, the discussion led to the identification of cognitions that might interfere with homework completion and ways to overcome them. Consideration of homework noncompliance in this manner reinforces the cognitive strategies described in Chapter 7. Third, the facilitators reinforced the rationale for doing homework and, in response to Dave's ambivalence, reinforced the rationale for the general cognitive approach to treating addictions. This reinforcement is necessary to ensure that facilitators and group members are operating under the same set of assumptions about the rationale for treatment. Finally, because it appeared that the brief intervention did not resolve Dave's ambivalence, the facilitators invited him to talk with them after the group session. During that individual meeting, the facilitators continued to express optimism that the CTAG would be helpful for Dave, but they also identified the need to modify homework assignments in a way that would be palatable to him.

On occasion, a group member misses one or more sessions, but then returns to a session with a completed homework assignment that is different than the one that was developed in the previous week's session. In such instances, facilitators take a brief moment to acknowledge the completion of homework, consolidate learning by asking the group member to explain how completing the homework made a difference in his or her life, and link it to the cognitive model and if possible, to the assignment that was completed by the majority of the group members.

CLOSURE

As stated previously, closure refers to the process of concluding or ending the group in a constructive, positive, effective manner for all group members. The method of closing a group session (or any psychotherapy session for that matter) will influence group members' thoughts and feelings about themselves between sessions, their likelihood of returning to treatment, their motivation to change, and their trust levels (for the group itself, other members, the facilitators, and more). A group that ends well may lead members to be hopeful, optimistic, motivated to change, and eager to return. A group that ends on a negative note may leave members depressed, fearful, dejected, likely to drop out, and vulnerable to a slip or relapse.

It is often more difficult to identify a need for closure in group therapy than it is in individual therapy. All group members bring their own unique style of expressing their struggles and concerns in the group. It is not uncommon for all but one or two members to feel good about a session, with one or two members feeling frustrated, unsettled, or unfulfilled. These members may hide their frustration for fear of judgment by other group members. Nevertheless, it is the facilitators' responsibility to try to identify members who need attention prior to ending a session. In many instances, facilitators can infer a group member's lack of closure by observing his or her facial expression, posture, and manner of participation in group discussion. Facilitators can also check in verbally with members who seem quiet, distant, and/or distressed.

In the following section, we describe general strategies for closure as well as ways to attempt closure in specific circumstances. We encourage facilitators to be mindful of the fact that, despite their best attempts, there will be times when some members do not achieve closure or leave the session with negative thoughts and feelings about the group.

Strategies for Closure

It is optimal to reserve the final 5–10 minutes of group for closure so that the main contents of the session can be summarized and members can leave feeling hopeful, motivated, and committed to change. Some questions for considering strategies for closure that facilitators can keep in mind as the session evolves are:

- What messages will group members take away from this session?
- How are group members likely to feel at the end of this session?
- Will all group members experience adequate closure? If not, who might need additional attention?
- How much time do we need to leave for the closure process?
- What procedures should we use to achieve closure for all members?

The actual strategy chosen will, to a large degree, depend on the content and process of the session. For example, if a session has gone well, and all group members are meeting their personal goals, they may not need a substantial block of time to get closure. A few minutes might be sufficient. When there is significant conflict between members, facilitators will leave a longer amount of time for closure so that these members and the rest of the group perceive that the conflict has been resolved and so that they feel safe to return. When facilitators sense that one or more members of the group did not gain adequate closure in the previous session, they might open the subsequent session with a question such as "Does anyone have any comments or reactions to the previous session?" Thus, if adequate closure is not gained in a particular session, all is not lost, as closure issues might be reintroduced as a bridge in the subsequent session from the previous session.

Closure When the Session Has Gone Well

When the session has gone smoothly, the facilitators might simply ask the group to reflect upon the topics discussed, the progress that group members are making, and the goals that members set for the next week. Facilitators can ask several questions that might prompt additional consolidation of learning, including

- "What have you learned in this session?"
- "What will you do differently as a result of this session?"
- "What healthy steps will you take this week?"
- "Is there anyone in the group who needs additional closure?"

These questions serve as a way to further engage group members in the therapeutic process, review session contents, consolidate learning, and begin to build a bridge from the contents of the current session to the contents of the subsequent session. Moreover, this approach to closure provides an opportunity for members to contemplate the manner in which all topics raised in session apply to their personal circumstances. Consider the following vignette:

FACILITATOR 1: We've covered a lot of ground today, and we only have a few minutes left. Who'd like to summarize what we've covered today?

ELLEN: I guess I can do that. It seemed that the main problem that the group discussed today is ways to recognize thinking that can get us into trouble. So we figured out ways to take a step back from that thinking.

FACILITATOR 2: Good, Ellen. (*looking to the group more generally*) And what were some of those specific ways to take a step back from unhelpful thinking?

ELLEN: Well, there were a bunch of ways to do that in my case. When I have thoughts about being all alone, I have to remember that those thoughts just lead me to wallow in my sadness and make me binge eat. They just make things worse. If I want more in my life, I have to actively do something about it.

BRIAN: And in my case it was to get some perspective when I get frustrated. I really have to keep my expectations in check and know that recovery from my gambling addiction will be a long, slow process.

MICHAEL: To me, it all goes back to the evidence. What's the evidence that really supports the way we're looking at a situation? And what's the evidence that does not fit with the way we're looking at a situation?

FACILITATOR 1: And what's the common theme here?

ALLISON: That we have to really examine our thinking before we take it as fact. Because if we take it as fact, all of a sudden if consumes us, and we don't even know for sure if it is true or not.

FACILITATOR 1: Dave, what do you think of all of this?

DAVE: I'm working on it.

FACILITATOR 1: (*winking at Dave*)

Closure When There Is Conflict

Facilitators can draw on cognitive and behavioral strategies to address conflict when it arises between group members. For example, if the facilitators infer from a group member's nonverbal behavior that he or she had a negative reaction to something another group member said, one of the facilitators might ask that member what was going through his or her mind at the moment and use Socratic questioning to reframe any cognitive distortions. Alternatively, facilitators may draw on the group's knowledge of assertiveness and communication skills to create an environment for the two members to address their differences. Not only would these strategies help to diffuse conflict by the end of the session and achieve adequate closure, but they also would model to the rest of the group healthy strategies for dealing with conflict in their own lives and facilitate interpersonal learning. Consider the following vignette, where some tension brewing between Michael and Dave erupted at the end of a session that was focused on continued discussion and practice of restructuring unhelpful situational cognitions:

FACILITATOR 1: I'd like to know what each of you will take away from today's group.

MICHAEL: This stuff is really helpful, guys. Trust me, it's saved my butt on more than one occasion.

DAVE: (*looking skeptical*) Maybe for *you* it's helpful. But you and I come from two different worlds.

MICHAEL: What's *that* supposed to mean?

DAVE: Come on, do I really have to say it? Your problem is that your fancy job sends you on fancy business trips and you get some action on the side? Sounds like a real problem to me!

(*Group members look uncomfortable.*)

MICHAEL: You know, I am really sick of your negative attitude in this group. The group seemed to gel a lot better before you came along. And ...

FACILITATOR 1: (*gently interrupting*) Let's slow down for a second here and take a look at what's going on. I can tell that both of you are irritated at one another.

MICHAEL: Well, where does he get the right to dismiss my problems?

DAVE: (*raising his voice*) Do you even have a clue what the rest of us go through? We can't afford to spend all that time doing the homework. We live paycheck to paycheck and have to make sure our lives don't fall apart.

ELLEN: I know things are tough for you, Dave. Even if you don't do your homework, I think you do a great job in group because you come almost every week, even when you have a lot of things going on at home. But that doesn't mean that Michael's problems aren't important, too.

FACILITATOR 1: I'd like to acknowledge that although this is uncomfortable, I commend both of you for saying what's on your mind rather than keeping it inside. I'm confident that we can resolve this in the remaining time. And my hope is that this will strengthen your bond to the group, rather than disrupt it, because you will learn that it is OK to deal with conflict head on and that it does not mean that the relationship is ruined.

DAVE: (*harrumphs*)

FACILITATOR 2: Who'd like to comment on what they see happening in this situation?

ALLISON: It seems like Dave thinks his problems are a lot worse than Michael's, and that doing the homework is easier said than done in his situation. But it also seems like Michael has a bit of an issue with Dave's attitude.

FACILITATOR 1: Great summary, Allison. So what have all of you learned in this group that might be useful in resolving this conflict?

MICHAEL: (*pausing for reflection*) You know what, I'm still angry at you for dismissing my problems, Dave, but I do apologize for bringing in a bunch of other issues, like your attitude and the group gelling and all.

DAVE: (*slight nod of head*)

FACILITATOR 2: Michael, you've highlighted an important communication strategy to keep in mind when there is conflict—sticking to the topic at hand and not bringing in other "baggage," as I like to call it.

ELLEN: I think, too, that it is understandable that Dave would be frustrated since he has a lot of things on his plate that make it difficult to use the coping skills. It's just important not to express that frustration as an attack toward someone else.

FACILITATOR 1: (*gently*) What do you think, Dave?

DAVE: (*sighing*) Yeah, I see what you mean.

FACILITATOR 1: Have there been other times in your life when that communication style has caused problems for you?

DAVE: (*laughing*) Yeah, once I got fired from a job because I told the owner that I'd like to crash into his precious little BMW.

(*Group laughs, and tension is beginning to decrease.*)

FACILITATOR 1: (*prompting Dave gently*) So how can you express what's on your mind in a way that is effective, rather than potentially dismissive of someone else?

DAVE: (*turning to Michael*) I do think we come from two different worlds. I would love to have all of what you have. But I guess we all have our own cards that we've been dealt.

MICHAEL: For what it's worth, I came from a background that is very different than the life I am living now. So I do think I might understand where you're coming from more than you think. And I'm really rooting for you, man. I just hope you'll give the group some credit because these skills really do work. I've seen it over and over with myself and with other group members.

FACILITATOR 1: (*seizing the opportunity for psychoeducation*) All of you are at different stages of change—some of you, like Michael, have been abstinent for a while and have a lot of experience in using cognitive and behavioral skills, whereas others of you are still using on occasion and/or have less experience in using the skills. That's actually a strength of our group—we are a diverse group, and we can learn from each other's experiences. The key is to have respect and tolerance for each other's differences. Remember the group rules?

ALLISON: I think the rules are very important. I don't think I'd feel comfortable sharing as much as I do without it.

BRIAN: And the other thing I appreciate about the group is that we're always welcomed back, even if we screw up.

DAVE: What if we do have a real problem with someone in the group, though?

FACILITATOR 2: That's a good question, Dave. I would encourage you to "choose your battles wisely," meaning that you might bring up these sorts of things after you've considered whether they would significantly help you, the other person, or the group in general. And when you do introduce this issue, I'd encourage you to choose your language carefully so that you are communicating respect to the other person. We've worked on this in the context of repairing relationships with family members, and it applies just as much here in group. In fact, this is a great place to practice these skills.

FACILITATOR 1: What are each of you going to take away from the manner in which we addressed this conflict between Michael and Dave?

MICHAEL: Like I said, it reminds me not to bring up my gripes with other issues that aren't relevant to the topic at hand.

DAVE: (*reluctantly*) I guess I need to make sure I'm not insulting the other person.

ALLISON: And it's important not to make assumptions about other people. It might be, Dave, that Michael is not as different than you as you think.

FACILITATOR 2: Is there anything from this discussion that you can translate to your own lives?

(*The group goes on to discuss the manner in which they can apply a "take-home" point from this conflict to manage a tense relationship in their own lives.*)

FACILITATOR 1: You've all done a great job in turning an interaction that began as uncomfortable for most people in the group into a learning experience. We'd like to be sure that everyone is settled before we leave here today. I'd like to check in with everyone regarding their mood, urges, and cravings.

Checking in with group members regarding their mood, urges, and cravings gives facilitators tangible evidence that adequate closure is being achieved. Facilitators can easily do this by asking group members to supply a number on a scale of 0–10 to indicate where they stand (i.e., 0 = *low mood or no urges and cravings*, 10 = *good mood or significant urges and cravings*). If group members' mood is generally good or at least neutral, and members report low levels of urges and cravings, then facilitators can have confidence that closure has been achieved. If one or more group members report low mood and/or a high level of urges and cravings, this is an indication that these individuals might require additional attention after the group. Some CTAG facilitators obtain these ratings after every group session, whereas others do so only if an event occurred during the session that had the potential to be unsettling.

When a Session Must End with Unsettled Members

Occasionally, it is simply not possible to end a group with all members feeling like they have adequate closure. In these cases, it is acceptable, or even essential, for the facilitators to ask those who need it to meet for a short time after the group or talk on the telephone to resolve problems and get closure. In our experience, we have found that group members are grateful when facilitators infer their need for closure and are able to resolve their concerns with just a small bit of extra attention.

In addition, it is important for facilitators to remember that the CTAG is not for everyone. Some members will not experience positive closure at the end of any CTAG session and will elect to complain bitterly or never return. Facilitators and other group members should expect this so that when it occurs, it is not shocking or upsetting. At times, it will even be necessary for the facilitators to address closure by telling a group member: "This type of group therapy might not be for you. I'd be happy to talk with you more about this, and if necessary, help you find a more appropriate form of treatment." By doing so, the facilitators are protecting other group members from walking away from sessions feeling perpetually frustrated by this member.

SUMMARY

Homework is an essential part of the CTAG because it encourages group members to practice the strategies learned in session in their own environments. Between-session practice increases the likelihood that group members will be able to successfully manage urges, cravings, and unpleasant mood states. Homework assignments are most successful when they follow logically from the group discussion, are developed collaboratively with group members and individually tailored to each person, are started in session, and are written down on a piece of paper. Facilitators always check in with group members about their homework assignments in the subsequent group session to reinforce the importance of between-session practice and to increase group members' accountability. Failure of any one group member to complete a homework assignment is viewed as useful information that allows the facilitators and that group member to continue to work collaboratively to ensure that the between-session work is relevant and helpful.

Because of the diversity of patients who participate in any one CTAG session, closure can take different forms. Sometimes it will take the form of a straightforward summary of the cognitive and behavioral strategies discussed in session. In other instances, it may be used to resolve a crisis that has emerged during the course of the session. Facilitators must accept that they will not always be able to achieve adequate closure due to time constraints, outbursts by members, or an inability to detect one or more member's distress. However, because CTAGs are flexible and structured in part on the basis of the needs of the particular members, alternative ways of achieving closure can be pursued, such as touching base with particular members outside of group, devoting the subsequent session to debriefing about a crisis that may have emerged in a previous session, or simply providing a bridge from the previous session to the subsequent session.

FORM 9.1. Homework Reminder Form

Date: _____

Today's homework assignment is: _____

_____
_____
_____
_____
_____
_____
_____

When will I commit to doing this assignment? _____

_____
_____
_____
_____
_____

Date: _____

This is what I learned from doing this assignment: _____

_____
_____
_____
_____
_____

FORM 9.2. Coping Skills Tracking Form

Date	Skill Used	Degree of Urges and Cravings (0 = *none*, 10 = *extreme*) PRE	Degree of Urges and Cravings (0 = *none*, 10 = *extreme*) POST

PART III SUMMARY AND INTEGRATION

INTRODUCTION TO PART III

Readers who have read to this point in the book have gained an understanding of the rationale for the development and implementation of the CTAG, the theory that underlies the treatment, the manner in which attention to group cohesiveness is balanced with attention to cognitive and behavioral change, and the specific activities that occur in the CTAG session components. Although readers undoubtedly have just as many questions as answers as they contemplate ways to implement the CTAG in their own clinical setting, we hope that this manual provides an overview of the fundamentals of this treatment and the manner in which they can apply to patients with a diverse array of addictive disorders.

The final chapter was written to pull the information presented in this volume into a coherent whole. In Chapter 10, readers will be reminded of the targets for treatment (included in the comprehensive cognitive model of addiction) and the manner in which the array of strategies described in this volume can address each of these targets. In addition, readers will begin to contemplate ways to handle instances in session that do not go as planned when they are faced with one or more challenging group members. Finally, readers will understand the value of anticipating a specific end date of treatment for each group member and the manner in which the concept of relapse prevention can be applied. After reading Part III, readers will have a framework for reflecting on the overall course of the CTAG for each individual group member and for the life of the group itself.

CHAPTER 10 | Conclusion

*Implementing the Cognitive
Therapy Addictions Group*

The cognitive therapy addictions group (CTAG) treatment approach was developed from a theoretical understanding of the cognitive and behavioral processes that lead to, maintain, and exacerbate addictive behavior (i.e., the comprehensive cognitive model of addiction; see Chapter 2) and the large body of empirical literature supporting the efficacy of cognitive behavioral therapy for the treatment of addictions and mood disturbance (see Chapter 1). It also incorporates practices that emerge from theory that speaks to group process (Yalom & Leszcz, 2005) and theory on patients' readiness for change (Prochaska & DiClemente, 2005). There are many characteristics of the CTAG that make it easy to implement in a wide range of settings. Because it is an open group, and because it targets an array of addictive behaviors, it can accommodate new members as they are referred; there is no need for new group members to wait until a new group is started or until there are enough people with a particular type of addiction to assemble a group. Thus, new group members will receive treatment in a timely manner, at a time when they are, perhaps, most vulnerable to relapse. Because the group targets cognitive and behavioral processes that are relevant to both addictive behavior and mood disturbance, it can accommodate "real-life" patients characterized by comorbidity and multiple life problems. We have seen CTAGs implemented successfully in intensive outpatient addiction treatment programs, outpatient medical centers, and even in private practices.

Despite this strength of the CTAG—its versatility—we also realize that clinicians who are in the process of learning about the cognitive therapy approach and, specifically, about CTAGs, might find the process of initiating an CTAG in their own facility a bit daunting. We have supervised clinicians who are concerned with whether they will be able to select the "best" strategies during the session, with whether they will be able to manage challenging group members, and with identifying the point at which a group member no longer needs the treatment. We address these concerns in this final chapter.

PUTTING IT ALL TOGETHER

On the one hand, the structure of each CTAG session is predictable—facilitators guide the group through introductions, education about the cognitive model, application of cognitive and behavioral strategies, review of previous homework and development of new homework, and closure. But on the other hand, the content and particular intervention strategy(ies) taught and practiced in each CTAG session are likely to be different for each group. There is no prescribed intervention that clinicians must implement in any one session. In fact, clinicians who first learn how to conduct CTAGs are often frustrated by the absence of a session-by-session guide!

We view this flexibility as another major strength of the CTAG. Facilitators and group members collaboratively decide on a focus of the group on the basis of the concerns raised by group members during introductions. The intervention or set of interventions (i.e., cognitive and behavioral strategies) that are implemented are selected on the basis of the case conceptualization and directly respond to the needs of group members. During the session, group members and facilitators discuss the rationale for the strategies; seasoned group members describe successes and challenges in using the strategies; group members identify creative ways to tailor the strategies to work in their own unique circumstances; and, in many instances, group members practice the strategies during the session. This flexible structure ensures that discussion is focused and productive, while, at the same time, it harnesses the power of the support that group members provide one another. It is expected that, by the end of the session, each group member will leave with something more than he or she had at the beginning of the session.

One of the most important lessons we have learned, then, is that all CTAG sessions are different. How could they not be different with so much diversity in the group? CTAG members have different addictions at different stages of the change process and therefore, the contents of sessions are inevitably diverse. At one point in time, the composition of the group may be 50% smokers, 20% problem drinkers, 20% overeaters, and 10% illicit drug users. At another point in time, or in another setting, the composition may be 60% illicit drug users, 35% problem drinkers, and 5% overeaters. As the patient composition changes, so does the content of the session and the use of time. As facilitators conduct CTAG sessions, it is important that they stay mindful of the manner in which the cognitive model of addiction applies to each group member, review participants' individual case conceptualizations as needed, and capture psychological processes that cut across the specific types of addictions. Interventions are selected strategically in order to target these psychological processes.

Figure 10.1 links CTAG intervention strategies with the components of the comprehensive cognitive model of addiction. As has been stated many times throughout this volume, facilitators need not be limited to the strategies that we describe—they can implement any strategy that targets the biopsychosocial processes included in the cognitive model of addiction and that follow from the conceptualization of group members' clinical presentations. However, this exhibit is a starting point for clinicians to consult as they are selecting a particular intervention to propose to group members.

Several points about the information contained in this exhibit deserve note. First, most of the strategies can be applied in the treatment of many of these psychological processes; conversely, each psychological process can be treated with an array of strategies. Cognitive restructuring, for example, can be applied to the evaluation of unhelpful addiction-related cognitions, cognitions associated with comorbid psychiatric disorders, cognitions that arise from problematic personality traits, and cognitions that have the potential to interfere with other goals of treatment such as the development of a social support network or engagement in meaningful activities. There is not necessarily a "right" or "wrong" strategy to use in the treatment of any of these psychological processes. Facilitators suggest a particular strategy on the basis of the degree to which it emerges from cognitive case conceptualization, the stages of change that characterize the group members, its ease of implementation, whether or not most group members have been exposed to the strategy in a previous session, and the degree to which the strategy might apply to other issues group members are experiencing. For instance, if several group members are not yet in the action stage of change and ambivalent about treatment, facilitators might select an easy-to-implement intervention so that group members can quickly see their benefit. A coping card would be an example of an easy-to-implement intervention because it can be created relatively quickly in session and can be used immediately in a time of distress. Conversely, if most group members are motivated for treatment and have had success in applying some of the easy-to-implement interventions, facilitators might suggest that the group focus on a more difficult-to-implement intervention. A Six-Column Thought Record would be an example of a more difficult-to-implement intervention because it requires practice, often over the course of more than one group session, to achieve its desired effect.

(text resumes on page 246)

PROXIMAL SITUATIONAL MODEL

Construct: **Activating stimuli**

Strategies:

- Use *distraction* when confronted with an activating stimulus.
- Use *imagery* to imagine the positive consequences of refraining from the addiction or the negative consequences of relapse.
- Use *imaginal rehearsal* to review the application of cognitive and behavioral strategies when confronted with an activating stimulus.
- Develop a *coping card* as a reminder of the cognitive and behavioral strategies to use when confronted with an activating stimulus.
- Conduct an *advantages–disadvantages analysis* to evaluate the consequences of relapse.
- Use *controlled breathing* to manage distress when confronted with an activating stimulus.
- Use *problem-solving skills* to make a healthy choice when confronted with an activating stimulus.

Construct: **Activation of expectancies**

Strategies:

- Use *cognitive restructuring* to develop an alternative response to outcome expectancies.
- Use *distraction* to turn one's attention away from outcome expectancies.
- Use *imagery* to imagine the positive consequences of refraining from the addiction or the negative consequences of relapse.
- Develop a *coping card* as a reminder of the cognitive and behavioral strategies to use when outcome expectancies are noticed.
- Conduct an *advantages–disadvantages analysis* to evaluate the consequences of relapse.

Construct: **Automatic thoughts**

Strategies:

- Use *cognitive restructuring* to develop an alternative response to unhelpful automatic thoughts.
- Use *distraction* to turn one's attention away from unhelpful automatic thoughts.
- Use *imagery* to imagine the positive consequences of refraining from the addiction or the negative consequences of relapse.
- Develop a *coping card* as a reminder of the cognitive and behavioral strategies to use when unhelpful automatic thoughts are noticed.
- Conduct an *advantages–disadvantages analysis* to evaluate the consequences of relapse.

(cont.)

FIGURE 10.1. Correspondence between the comprehensive cognitive model of addiction and CTAG intervention strategies.

Construct: **Urges and cravings**

Strategies:

- Use *distraction* to turn one's attention away from urges and cravings.
- Use *imagery* to imagine the positive consequences of refraining from the addiction or the negative consequences of relapse.
- Use *imaginal rehearsal* to review the application of cognitive and behavioral strategies to manage the fallout from relapse.
- Develop a *coping card* as a reminder of the cognitive and behavioral strategies to use when urges and cravings are noticed.
- Conduct an *advantages–disadvantages analysis* to evaluate the consequences of relapse.
- Use *controlled breathing* to manage distress associated with urges and cravings.
- Use *problem-solving skills* to make a healthy choice when dealing with urges and cravings.

Construct: **Facilitating thoughts**

Strategies:

- Use *cognitive restructuring* to develop an alternative response to facilitating thoughts.
- Use *distraction* to turn one's attention away from facilitating thoughts.
- Use *imagery* to imagine the positive consequences of refraining from the addiction or the negative consequences of relapse.
- Develop a *coping card* as a reminder of the cognitive and behavioral strategies to use when facilitating thoughts are noticed.
- Conduct an *advantages–disadvantages analysis* to evaluate the consequences of relapse.

Construct: **Instrumental strategies**

Strategies:

- Conduct an *advantages–disadvantages analysis* to evaluate the consequences of relapse.
- Use *problem-solving skills* to make a healthy choice when initiating instrumental strategies.

Construct: **Continued use or relapse**

Strategies:

- Use *imagery* to imagine the positive consequences of refraining from the addiction or the negative consequences of relapse.
- Conduct an *advantages–disadvantages analysis* to evaluate the consequences of relapse.
- Use *problem-solving skills* to make a healthy choice after continuing to engage in addictive behavior.

(cont.)

FIGURE 10.1. *(cont.)*

Construct: **Self-efficacy**

Strategies:

- Use *cognitive restructuring* to develop an alternative response to thoughts associated with low self-efficacy.
- Develop a *coping card* as a reminder of previous successes.
- *Practice* using the cognitive and behavioral strategies over and over.

Construct: **Attentional bias, attentional fixation, and perceived availability**

Strategy:

- Use *distraction* to turn one's attention away from addiction-related cues.

DISTAL BACKGROUND MODEL

Construct: **Genetic predisposition**

Strategies:

- Use *psychoeducation* to help group members to understand the manner in which their genetic predisposition makes them vulnerable to addictive behavior and psychiatric disorders.
- Develop a *relapse prevention plan* that outlines ways to cope in light of these vulnerabilities.

Construct: **Personality traits**

Strategies:

- Use *cognitive restructuring* to develop an alternative response to unhelpful thoughts associated with a problematic personality trait.
- Develop a *coping card* as a reminder of the cognitive and behavioral strategies to use when unhelpful cognitions or behaviors associated with the personality trait are noticed.
- Conduct an *advantages–disadvantages analysis* to evaluate the consequences of engaging in risky behavior associated with a problematic personality trait.

Construct: **Psychiatric disorder**

Strategies:

- Use *cognitive restructuring* to develop an alternative response to unhelpful thoughts associated with the psychiatric disorder.
- Develop a *coping card* as a reminder of the cognitive and behavioral strategies to use when unhelpful cognitions or behaviors associated with the psychiatric disorder are noticed.
- Conduct an *advantages–disadvantages analysis* to evaluate the consequences of engaging in risky behavior associated with a psychiatric disorder.

(cont.)

FIGURE 10.1. *(cont.)*

- Use *activity monitoring and scheduling* to increase engagement in meaningful activities (an antidote for depression).
- Use *controlled breathing* to manage distress associated with a psychiatric disorder.
- Use *muscle relaxation* to manage distress associated with a psychiatric disorder.
- Use *problem-solving skills* to make a healthy choice when dealing with the effects of a psychiatric disorder.
- Use *psychoeducation* to help group members understand the importance of leading a healthy lifestyle (e.g., regular meals, sleep) in managing symptoms of a psychiatric disorder.
- *Monitor* aspects of a healthy lifestyle (e.g., regular meals, sleep) in order to identify places to make adjustments.

Construct: **Early life experiences**

Strategies:

- Use *psychoeducation* to help group members understand the manner in which their early life experiences make them vulnerable to addictive behavior and psychiatric disorders.
- Develop a *relapse prevention plan* that outlines ways to cope in light of these vulnerabilities.

Construct: **Exposure to and experimentation with addictions**

Strategies:

- Use *psychoeducation* to help group members to understand the manner in which exposure to and experimentation with addictions makes them vulnerable to addictive behavior.
- Develop a *relapse prevention plan* that outlines ways to cope in light of these vulnerabilities.

Construct: **Social support network**

Strategies:

- Use *cognitive restructuring* to develop an alternative response to unhelpful cognitions that interfere with developing or utilizing one's social support network.
- Develop a *coping card* as a reminder of the cognitive and behavioral strategies to use when unhelpful cognitions or behaviors that interfere with developing or utilizing one's social support network are noticed.
- Conduct an *advantages–disadvantages analysis* to evaluate relationship choices.
- *Participate in shared activities* with people in social support network who do not engage in addictive behavior.
- Implement *effective verbal, nonverbal, and active listening communication skills* to enhance relationships with people who do not engage in addictive behavior.
- Identify ways to *meet new people* who do not engage in addictive behavior in order to build one's social support network.

(cont.)

FIGURE 10.1. *(cont.)*

Construct: **Meaningful activities**

Strategies:
- Use *cognitive restructuring* to develop an alternative response to unhelpful thoughts that interfere with engaging in meaningful activities.
- Develop a *coping card* as a reminder of the cognitive and behavioral strategies to use when unhelpful cognitions or behaviors that interfere with engaging in meaningful activities are noticed.
- Conduct an *advantages–disadvantages analysis* to evaluate choices about activities to pursue.
- Use *activity monitoring and scheduling* to increase the frequency of engagement in meaningful activities.

Construct: **Basic beliefs**

Strategies:
- Use *cognitive restructuring* to develop an alternative response to unhelpful basic beliefs.
- Use the *cognitive continuum* to evaluate and modify all-or-nothing basic beliefs (e.g., "I am a failure").
- Implement a *behavioral experiment* to test aspects of the basic belief.
- Develop a *coping card* as a reminder of evidence that supports a new, healthier basic belief.
- Conduct an *advantages–disadvantages analysis* to evaluate the consequences of holding onto an unhelpful basic belief.

Construct: **Addiction-related beliefs**

Strategies:
- Use *cognitive restructuring* to develop an alternative response to unhelpful addiction-related beliefs.
- Develop *control beliefs* to counteract the addiction-related beliefs.
- Develop a *coping card* as a reminder of evidence that supports a control belief.
- Conduct an *advantages–disadvantages analysis* to evaluate the consequences of holding onto an unhelpful addiction-related belief.

FIGURE 10.1. *(cont.)*

Second, the strategies described in this volume need not be applied *only* in the manner in which we presented them. They can be creatively adapted to meet the needs of the group. A case in point is the advantages–disadvantages analysis. Earlier in the volume, we described the manner in which this strategy is applied when group members are deciding whether or not to engage in addictive behavior, or in instances in which they are deciding whether to put themselves in a position where they will encounter an activating stimulus. However, in Figure 10.1, we also include the advantages–disadvantages analysis as a strategy that has the potential to be useful in developing a social support network, engaging in meaningful activities, and modifying basic and addiction-related beliefs. Facilitators can work with group members to evaluate the advantages and disadvantages of repairing an existing relationship or starting a new relationship, of overcoming inertia and procrastination as group members begin to engage in more meaningful activities, and of holding on to certain beliefs that keep group members "stuck" in self-defeating behavioral patterns. Thus, we encourage facilitators to take the time to understand the principles that underlie these intervention strategies, as knowledge of these principles will allow the creative and flexible application of them in session.

Third, some of the constructs in the cognitive model of addiction cannot be modified, such as group members' genetic predispositions, the early experiences they had during their formative years, or early exposure to and experimentation with addictive behavior. Nevertheless, these constructs can still inform treatment. It is often helpful for facilitators to provide psychoeducation about the manner in which these vulnerabilities affect the likelihood of relapse and mood disturbance. Many group members report tremendous guilt about their addictive behavior and mood disturbance, and psychoeducation about these vulnerabilities helps these group members to see that it is understandable that they have struggled in light of their histories. Moreover, knowledge of these vulnerabilities allows group members to put together a relapse prevention plan, such that they identify triggers that are relevant in light of these vulnerabilities and plan, proactively, for ways to cope in the face of those triggers. For example, Dave likely had a genetic vulnerability for alcohol and drug abuse, given that his father and many other family members had a history of these addictions. After participating in the group for several months, Dave admitted that he realized that this vulnerability would make it particularly difficult for him to continue to drink in a controlled manner. He changed his goal to abstinence, and he acknowledged that just being in the presence of alcohol (e.g., spending time with friends who continue to drink heavily) would be likely to serve as a trigger.

CHALLENGING GROUP MEMBERS

According to Bieling et al. (2006), in almost every group they conduct, facilitators have at least one challenging group member. Thus, it is wise for facilitators to have the expectation that they will need to manage a challenging group member in any one session. Challenging group members can come in many forms—they can talk endlessly and monopolize the discussion, they can have the opposite problem and say very little, they can engage in behavior that has the potential to disrupt the session (e.g., arriving late, interrupting others), they can provide a great amount of advice to others without talking about themselves, or they can present with an angry or resistant stance if they perceive that they are not attending of their own accord (Bieling et al., 2006; L. C. Sobell & Sobell, 2011).

In managing these challenging group members, facilitators keep in mind that the CTAG is an active treatment that is most effective when there is a balance between the facilitators modeling, teaching, and guiding, and the group members providing support and feedback to one another. This means that, when facilitators notice the potential for a problem associated with the interactional style of a challenging group member, they address it at that time, rather than letting it continue; however, active intervention to manage a challenging group member does not always necessitate that the facilitators take the lead in providing feedback and redirecting the group. Instead, facilitators might ask group members for feedback on how they are reacting to the challenging group member's comments or behavior, or whether they have any suggestions for the challenging group member.

Whenever possible, an intervention to manage a challenging group member should model the cognitive and behavioral strategies that are taught and practiced in the group. Think back to the conflict between Michael and Dave that emerged as the group was working toward closure in Chapter 9. In most sessions, Dave presented as a challenge to the facilitators because he often had a negative attitude about the cognitive and behavioral strategies being discussed. In this session, he was particularly challenging because he expressed disdain toward Michael, implying that Michael had it easier than the other group members. The facilitators took this opportunity to work with the group to identify communication skills that could have been used to work through their differences more effectively and consider the manner in which these skills would be useful for group members to keep in mind in their own lives. It was also pointed out in this vignette that Dave was making the assumption that Michael's background was much different than his. The facilitators also could have used cognitive strategies for helping Dave see that he was making an assumption, taking that assumption as fact, and allowing that assumption to affect his feelings about and behavior toward Michael. Such an illustration would reinforce the association between cognition, emotion, and behavior, and remind the group that it is important to notice their assumptions and check them out before accepting them as fact.

Figure 10.2 displays examples of some typical ways that facilitators can manage challenging group members and the tension or conflict that results from their behavior. Many of these strategies involve a short, one- or two-sentence summary statement by one of the facilitators, often that comments on the process of what is happening in the discussion and/or acknowledges affect, and invites other group members to share their own

- When a group member is dominating the discussion: *It sounds like this has been a difficult week for you, and there is a lot going on. Let's check in and hear what is happening with the other group members so that we can decide, as a group, the best way to go about addressing our difficulties.*

- When a group member has said something offensive or off-putting: *I'm noticing some tension here. Let's talk about it. How do other people feel about what _____ just said?*

- When a group member contributes very little: *We've just heard about some of the difficulties that others have experienced in the past week. I know/imagine you have had similar experiences. What suggestions might you have for dealing with these difficulties?*

- When a group member discloses very personal information that has the potential to be uncomfortable for others: *Let's hear from the others. What might it feel like to be in that situation?*

- When a group member readily gives advice to others but does not talk about him- or herself: *You seem to have a lot of wisdom and experience that can be applied to others. How might you apply this to managing your own addiction?*

- When a group member demonstrates a negative attitude toward treatment: *It sounds as if you're not convinced that this treatment will be helpful. Has anyone else had a similar reaction? How did you work through it?*

- When the group itself is getting activated and many people are speaking at once: *This is a useful discussion, but I'm noticing that many people are talking at once. How can we simultaneously respect one another and hear what others have to say while also getting our own needs met?*

FIGURE 10.2. Strategies for managing challenging group members. Sources: Bieling et al. (2006); L. C. Sobell and Sobell (2011).

reactions or make suggestions. In other words, facilitators gently intervene and turn the challenging moment into a learning opportunity for the entire group. Of course, there are instances in which facilitators skillfully use these approaches, and one or more challenging group members' problematic behavior does not subside. In these instances, it is reasonable to address the problem with the group member outside of session.

THE END OF TREATMENT

The decision to end participation in the CTAG is an individualized one for each group member. Some group members decide to discontinue treatment when they have reached the goals that they set for themselves at the beginning of their participation in group, such as sustained abstinence. Other group members have reached their goals but choose to continue participation in the CTAG; these group members are regarded as being in the maintenance stage of change, and they continue to attend sessions to hone their cognitive and behavioral coping skills and remain focused on recovery. Of course, there are other group members who discontinue treatment without having reached their goals. There are many reasons for this—some of these individuals decide that the cognitive approach is not a good fit for them, whereas others are ambivalent about treatment and ultimately decide to continue to engage in addictive behavior.

It is easy for group members who have reached their goals to drift off in their attendance, attending fewer and fewer sessions until they eventually attend none at all. However, we strongly recommend that facilitators work with group members to plan for their final session so that it can be a learning experience for all (cf. Bernard et al., 2008). In that final session, the group can acknowledge the gains that the group member has made, thereby increasing that group member's self-efficacy and instilling hope in newer group members that change is possible. A final session also allows for the group member to consolidate his or her learning and for other group members to reaffirm their commitment to their individual goals. It provides a context for the group to revisit the important topic of relapse and for the departing group member to commit to a relapse prevention plan. Moreover, it gives the opportunity for the facilitators to communicate that the group member is welcome back whenever he or she perceives there is a need for a review. In the following vignette, Michael has decided to discontinue participation in the group after attending sessions for 13 months and achieving sustained abstinence during that time. The group members agreed to focus their cognitive behavioral work on the topic of relapse:

FACILITATOR 1: Michael, any words of wisdom for the other group members regarding the topic of relapse?

MICHAEL: I think we're all going to be prone to relapse for the rest of our lives. Addictions are just so powerful. But, take it from me, it really helps to keep practicing what we learn in group.

ALLISON: I can't tell you how much I've learned from you, Michael. Your success has really shown me that I can beat my addiction if I put my mind to it.

BRIAN: Yeah, I'm gonna make it my mission to be sitting where you're sitting 6 months from now.

MICHAEL: Thanks, guys, I really appreciate it. But I honestly think that we *all* deserve credit because we all help each other out and figure out the best ways to apply the strategies.

FACILITATOR 2: (*focusing on consolidating learning*) Michael, would you be willing to share the most important take-home points that you're leaving the group with?

MICHAEL: *(taking a deep breath)* That's a tough one, there are so many.

FACILITATOR 2: In my experience, I have found that when people are ready to leave the group, it is very helpful to have a written relapse prevention plan so that they have the most helpful cognitive and behavioral strategies in one place, which allows for easy consultation. The plan also includes reminders of indicators that getting additional help might be a good idea. Would you be willing to put together a plan like that?

MICHAEL: I think that's a good idea. I'm actually a little nervous about what it will be like without coming to the group.

FACILITATOR 2: *(turning to the rest of the group)* And this exercise doesn't just have to be for people who are getting ready to leave the group. A relapse prevention plan is helpful no matter where in the process of recovery you are, as it reminds you of triggers and ways to manage them. Would everyone else be willing to work on this, as well?

(Group members nod their heads, and Facilitator 1 distributes the handout presented in Form 10.1 [at the end of the chapter].)

FACILITATOR 1: *(after giving group members some time to complete the form)* Let's see what all of you have come up with. What are some of the triggers that you notice, along with strategies to handle those triggers?

ELLEN: Watching sappy movies on TV does not help me whatsoever. I know I need to do things that are better for myself, like calling my daughter, now that we're talking again, or quilting. I've finally lost some weight—8 pounds!

(Group members give Ellen a thumbs up.)

ELLEN: I don't want to mess up my hard work.

BRIAN: Having extra money is most definitely my biggest trigger. Whenever I come into extra money, I now immediately give it to my wife. She said she's willing to stay and try to work things out if I agreed to this plan.

ELLEN: Oh, Brian, that's wonderful!

ALLISON: Yeah, that's great! For me, I have lots of triggers, but the biggest one is knowing my husband and mother-in-law are smoking in the house. That's when I have the most facilitating thoughts. So I have to remember the alternative response—smoking just one takes me farther away from the goals I've set for myself, and it's not worth it to jeopardize those goals. And then I go and call one of my friends from work, since I've gotten closer to them.

FACILITATOR 2: (*eying Dave*) Dave?

DAVE: I just have to accept that I can't be around it. If alcohol is near me, I'll drink it. If weed is around me, I'll smoke it.

FACILITATOR 2: So being in the presence of a substance is the trigger. Say you are at a barbeque, and some of the guests are drinking beers. How would you handle that trigger?

DAVE: I need to get away from them, and fast. (*thinking for a moment*) I think in this case, I could go and help at the grill. Now that it's summer, I've become Chef Barbeque.

(*Group chuckles.*)

FACILITATOR 2: So what type of coping strategy is that, Dave?

DAVE: I guess that would be distraction?

FACILITATOR 2: You got it.... And how about you, Michael? We want to make sure your plan is complete when you leave here. For the rest of you, we can revisit these plans periodically and add to them or modify them.

MICHAEL: I've noticed three triggers. Being out of town, having that freedom, that's number one. I think what's most helpful for that is the advantages–disadvantages analysis. The other triggers are talking with a coworker or a client I find very attractive, or being invited to go to a strip club after work. In those cases, I imagine my wife's reaction and the consequences if she were to find out that I slipped. But I also imagine positives, like doing things as a family again, and being there for my children for the little things, like tucking them in at night, and the bigger things, like their school plays and family vacations.

ALLISON: Wow, sounds like you've covered everything, Michael.

The facilitators continued on to stimulate a discussion of the manner in which other cognitive and behavioral strategies would apply in managing their addictive behavior and addressing related problems, such as mood disturbance and relationship distress. They also guided discussion in the identification of warning signs that might signal that the group members are vulnerable to a relapse and what to do when those warning signs are noticed. Examples of actions group members can take include (1) attending a CTAG session, (2) attending an extra 12-step meeting, (3) reaching out for help from a trusted close other, (4) telling their psychiatrist or therapist, and (5) calling a 24-hour addiction hotline. In cases in which group members indicated that they would reach out to or call someone, the specific name of the individual was provided, as well as his or her phone number, so all of the necessary information was on the sheet of paper. When group members indicated they would call a hotline, the specific number of the hotline was recorded. This discussion took the majority of the time in session, and in the last 10 minutes of the group, the facilitators moved toward closure:

> FACILITATOR 1: You've all done very important work today. In fact, the relapse prevention plan may be the most important piece of paper you will leave here with during the time in which you participate in the group.
>
> MICHAEL: Thanks, everyone, for your support throughout the past months, as well as your help today in making sure I have all of this information in one place. Even though I'm going to have to watch out for triggers, I really think I've overcome my addiction.
>
> ELLEN: It has really been so nice getting to know you. My road to recovery has been pretty bumpy, but if you could do it, I know I can too, if I put my mind to it.
>
> DAVE: Yeah, and I guess I need to say thanks for putting up with me over the past several months.
>
> MICHAEL: (acknowledging Dave's way of saying good-bye and ending their relationship on a positive note by reaching across the table and shaking his hand) I appreciate it, Dave. I really do. And you know what, I've seen a lot of changes in you. I really do wish you all the best.
>
> DAVE: (nodding his head toward Michael and smiling)
>
> FACILITATOR 1: Michael, the door is always open if you'd like to come back. And it doesn't have to be a full-on relapse that brings you back. If, in a few months, you'd like to attend a session to brush up on your strategies, just let me know.
>
> MICHAEL: Will do. I really appreciate that.

CONCLUDING THOUGHTS

Clinical work with patients with addictions can be challenging and difficult; yet it is incredibly rewarding when these patients begin to make positive changes in their lives, make progress toward meeting their goals, and exhibit evidence that they can successfully apply the cognitive and behavioral strategies described in this volume. The open nature of the CTAG allows for much stimulation and diversity, providing a forum for numerous learning experiences to arise from group interactions, and practice in applying cognitive and behavioral strategies. Because group interventions are more cost-effective than individual interventions (Morrison, 2001; L. C. Sobell et al., 2009), it is likely that they will be the treatment of choice in the future (L. C. Sobell & Sobell, 2011). Thus, we expect to see an increasing number of CTAGs implemented in a variety of settings, from those that specialize in addictions treatment to those that, more generally, serve people with a variety of mental health problems. Many group members have expressed gratitude for the opportunity to participate in the CTAG, noting that, for the first time in their lives, they have developed specific coping strategies that make a difference for them. As a result, group members develop a renewed sense of hope and optimism for treatment success and for the possibility of having a significantly improved quality of life. We eagerly await for continued research on the efficacy and effectiveness of this treatment package and dissemination to a diverse array of clinical settings.

FORM 10.1. Relapse Prevention Plan

Trigger	Strategy for handling the trigger

Other helpful strategy	What it is helpful for

Warning signs that I might need extra help in order not to relapse: _____

_____

_____

_____

_____

What will I do if I notice one or more of these warning signs? _____

_____

_____

_____

_____

References

Addis, M. E., & Jacobson, N. S. (2000). A closer look at the treatment rationale and homework compliance in cognitive-behavioral therapy for depression. *Cognitive Therapy and Research, 24*, 313–326.

American Psychiatric Association. (2000). *Diagnostic and statistical manual of mental disorders* (4th ed., text rev.). Washington, DC: Author.

American Psychiatric Association. (2010). *DSM-5 development: Substance use and addictive disorders.* Retrieved from *http://dsm5.org/proposedrevision/ Pages/SubstanceUseandAddictiveDisorders.aspx.*

American Society of Addiction Medicine. (n.d.) *About ASAM.* Retrieved from *www.asam.org/About.html.*

Anda, R. F., Whitfield, C. L., Felitti, V. J., Chapman, D., Edwards, V. J., Dube, S. R., et al. (2002). Adverse childhood experiences, alcoholic parents, and later risks of alcoholism and depression. *Psychiatric Services, 53*, 1001–1009.

Bandura, A. (1977). Self-efficacy: Toward a unifying theory of behavior change. *Psychological Review, 84*, 191–215.

Beck, A. T. (1976). *Cognitive therapy and the emotional disorders.* Oxford, UK: International Universities Press.

Beck, A. T. (1999). *Prisoners of hate: The cognitive basis of anger, hostility, and violence.* New York: HarperCollins.

Beck, A. T., & Alford, B. A. (2009). *Depression: Causes and treatment* (2nd ed.). Philadelphia: University of Pennsylvania Press.

Beck, A. T., & Emery, G. (2005). *Anxiety disorders and phobias: A cognitive perspective.* New York: Basic Books.

Beck, A. T., Freeman, A., Davis, D. D., & Associates. (2004). *Cognitive therapy of personality disorders* (2nd ed.). New York: Guilford Press.

Beck, A. T., Rush, A. J., Shaw, B. F., & Emery, G. (1979). *Cognitive therapy of depression.* New York: Guilford Press.

Beck, A. T., Wright, F. D., Newman, C. F., & Liese, B. S. (1993). *Cognitive therapy of substance abuse.* New York: Guilford Press.

Beck, J. S. (2005). *Cognitive therapy for challenging problems: What to do when the basics don't work.* New York: Guilford Press.

Beck, J. S. (2011). *Cognitive behavior therapy: Basics and beyond* (2nd ed.). New York: Guilford Press.

Bernard, H., Burlingame, G., Flores, P., Greene, L., Joyce, A., Kobos, J. C., et al. (2008). Clinical practice guidelines for group psychotherapy. *International Journal of Group Psychotherapy, 58*, 455–542.

Bieling, P. J., McCabe, M. E., & Antony, M. M. (2006). *Cognitive-behavioral therapy in groups*. New York: Guilford Press.

Bourne, E. J. (2010). *The anxiety and phobia workbook* (5th ed.). Oakland, CA: New Harbinger.

Brandon, T., Herzog, T., Irvin, J., & Gwaltney, C. (2004). Cognitive and social learning models of drug dependence: Implications for the assessment of tobacco dependence in adolescents. *Addiction, 99*(Suppl. 1), 51–77.

Brandon, T. H., & Baker, T. B. (1991). The Smoking Consequences Questionnaire: The subjective utility of smoking in college students. *Psychological Assessment: A Journal of Consulting and Clinical Psychology, 3*, 484–491.

Brenner, V. (1997). Psychology of computer use: VLVII: Parameters of Internet use, abuse, and addiction: The first 90 dates of the Internet Usage Survey. *Psychological Reports, 80*, 879–882.

Breslau, N., Johnson, E. O., Hiripi, E., & Kessler, R. (2001). Nicotine dependence in the United States. *Archives of General Psychiatry, 58*, 810–816.

Brown, R. F. (1989). Relapses from a gambling perspective. In M. Gossop (Ed.), *Relapse and addictive behaviour* (pp. 107–132). New York: Tavistock/Routledge.

Bruce, G., & Jones, B. T. (2006). Methods, measures, and findings of attentional bias in substance use, abuse, and dependence. In R. W. Wiers & A. W. Stacy (Eds.), *Handbook of implicit cognition and addictions* (pp. 135–149). Thousand Oaks, CA: Sage.

Burlingame, G. M., Fuhriman, A., & Johnson, J. E. (2002). Cohesion in group psychotherapy. In J. C. Norcross (Ed.), *Psychotherapy relationships that work* (pp. 71–87). New York: Oxford University Press.

Burlingame, G. M., McClendon, D. T., & Alonso, J. (2011). Cohesion in group therapy. *Psychotherapy, 48*, 34–42.

Burns, D. D. (1980). *Feeling good: The new mood therapy*. New York: Morrow.

Burns, D. D. (1999). *The feeling good handbook* (rev. ed.). New York: Plume/Penguin Books.

Butler, A. C., Chapman, J. E., Forman, E. M., & Beck, A. T. (2006). The empirical status of cognitive-behavioral therapy: A review of meta-analyses. *Clinical Psychology Review, 26*, 17–31.

Carroll, K. M., Nich, C., Ball, S. A., McCance-Katz, E. F., Frankforter, T. F., & Rounsaville, B. J. (2000). One-year follow-up of disulfiram and psychotherapy for cocaine-alcohol abusers: Sustained effects of treatment. *Addiction, 95*, 1335–1349.

Carroll, K. M., Rounsaville, B. J., Nich, C., Gordon, L. T., Wirtz, P. W., & Gawin, F. H. (1994). One year follow-up of psychotherapy and pharmacotherapy for cocaine dependence: Delayed emergence of psychotherapy effects. *Archives of General Psychiatry, 51*, 989–997.

Cassin, S. E., & von Ranson, K. M. (2007). Is binge eating experienced as an addiction? *Appetite, 49,* 687–690.

Centers for Disease Control and Prevention. (2008). Smoking-attributable mortality, years of potential life lost, and productivity losses—United States, 2000–2004. *Morbidity and Mortality Weekly Report, 57,* 1226–1228. Retrieved from *www.cdc.gov/mmwr/preview/mmwrhtml/mm5745a3.htm.*

Chen, G. (2010). Gender differences in sense of coherence, perceived social support, and negative emotions among drug-abstinent Israeli inmates. *International Journal of Offender Therapy and Comparative Criminology, 54,* 937–958.

Clark, D. A., & Beck, A. T. (2010). *Cognitive therapy of anxiety disorders: Science and practice.* New York: Guilford Press.

Clark, D. M. (1986). A cognitive approach to panic. *Behaviour Research and Therapy, 24,* 461–470.

Cohen, S., Lichtenstein, E., Prochaska, J. O., Rossi, J. S., Gritz, E. R., & Carr, C. R. (1989). Debunking myths about self-quitting: Evidence from 10 prospective studies of persons who attempted to quit smoking by themselves. *American Psychologist, 44,* 1355–1365.

Collins, R. L. (2005). Relapse prevention for eating disorders and obesity. In G. A. Marlatt & D. M. Donovan (Eds.), *Relapse prevention: Maintenance strategies in the treatment of addictive behaviors* (2nd ed., pp. 248–275). New York: Guilford Press.

Cooper, A., Delmonico, D. L., & Burg, R. (2000). Cybersex users, abusers, and compulsives: New findings and implications. *Sexual Addiction and Compulsivity, 7,* 5–29.

Cooper, A., Scherer, C., Boies, S. C., & Gordon, B. (1999). Sexuality on the Internet: From sexual exploration to pathological expression. *Professional Psychology: Research and Practice, 30,* 154–164.

Craske, M. G., & Barlow, D. H. (2006). *Mastery of your anxiety and panic: Therapist guide* (3rd ed.). New York: Oxford University Press.

Craske, M. G., & Barlow, D. H. (2008). Panic disorder and agoraphobia. In D. H. Barlow (Ed.), *Clinical handbook of psychological disorders: A step-by-step treatment manual* (4th ed., pp. 1–64). New York: Guilford Press.

Crits-Christoph, P., Siqueland, L., Blaine, J., Frank, A., Luborsky, L., Onken, L. S., et al. (1999). Psychosocial treatments for cocaine dependence: National Institute on Drug Abuse Collaborative Cocaine Treatment Study. *Archives of General Psychiatry, 56,* 493–502.

Davis, C. A., Levitan, R. D., Reid, C., Carter, J. C., Kaplan, A. S., Patte, K. A., et al. (2009). Dopamine for "wanting" and opioids for "liking": A comparison of obese adults with and without binge eating. *Obesity, 17,* 1220–1225.

Degenhardt, L., Chiu, W-T., Sampson, N., Kessler, R. C., Anthony, J. C., Angermeyer, M., et al. (2008). Toward a global view of alcohol, tobacco, cannabis, and cocaine use: Findings from the WHO World Mental Health Surveys. *PLoS Medicine, 5,* 1–14.

Des Jarlais, D. (1995). Harm reduction: A framework for incorporating science into drug policy. *American Journal of Public Health, 85,* 10–12.

DiClemente, C. C., & Prochaska, J. O. (1998). Toward a comprehensive, theoretical model of change: Stages of change and addictive behaviors. In W. R. Miller & N. Heather (Eds.), *Treating addictive behaviors* (2nd ed., pp. 3–24). New York: Plenum Press.

Dom, G., D'haene, P., Hulstijn, W., & Sabbe, B. (2006). Impulsivity in abstinent early- and late-onset alcoholics: Differences in self-report measures and a discounting task. *Addiction, 101,* 50–59.

Dougherty, D. M., Mathias, C. W., Marsh-Richard, D. M., Furr, R., Nouvion, S. O., & Dawes, M. A. (2009). Distinctions in behavioral impulsivity: Implications for substance abuse research. *Addictive Disorders and Their Treatment, 8,* 61–73.

Dunn, P. C. (2000). The stages and processes of change model: Implications for social work ATOD practice. In A. A. Abbott (Ed.), *Alcohol, tobacco, and other drugs: Challenging myths, assessing theories, individualizing interventions* (pp. 111–143). Washington, DC: NASW Press.

Dutra, L., Stathopoulou, G., Basden, S. L., Leyro, T. M., Powers, M. B., & Otto, M. W. (2008). A meta-analytic review of psychosocial interventions for substance use disorders. *American Journal of Psychiatry, 165,* 179–187.

D'Zurilla, T. J., & Nezu, A. M. (2007). *Problem-solving therapy: A positive approach to clinical intervention* (3rd ed.). New York: Springer.

Enticott, P. G., & Ogloff, J. P. (2006). Elucidation of impulsivity. *Australian Psychologist, 41,* 3–14.

Epstein, D. E., Hawkins, W. E., Covi, L., Umbricht, A., & Preston, K. L. (2003). Cognitive behavioral therapy plus contingency management for cocaine use: Findings during treatment and across 12-month follow-up. *Psychology of Addictive Behavior, 17,* 73–82.

Field, M., & Cox, W. M. (2008). Attentional bias in addictive behaviors: A review of its development, causes, and consequences. *Drug and Alcohol Dependence, 97,* 1–20.

Field, M., & Eastwood, B. (2005). Experimental manipulation of attentional bias increases the motivation to drink alcohol. *Psychopharmacology, 183,* 350–357.

Field, M., Mogg, K., & Bradley, B. P. (2006). Attention to drug-related cues in drug abuse and addiction: Component processes. In R. W. Wiers & A. W. Stacy (Eds.), *Handbook of implicit cognition and addictions* (pp. 151–163). Thousand Oaks, CA: Sage.

First, M. B., Spitzer, R. L., Gibbon, M., & Williams, J. B. W. (2002). *Structured Clinical Interview for DSM-IV-TR Axis I Disorders, research version, patient edition (SCID-I/P).* New York: Biometrics Research, New York State Psychiatric Institute.

Flores, P. J. (2007). *Group psychotherapy with addicted populations: An integration of twelve-step and psychodynamic theory.* New York: Routledge.

Folkman, S., & Moskowitz, J. (2004). Coping: Pitfalls and promise. *Annual Review of Psychology, 55,* 745–774.

Forbes, E. E., Brown, S. M., Kimak, M., Ferrell, R. E., Manuck, S. B., & Hariri, A. R. (2009). Genetic variation in components of dopamine neurotransmission impacts ventral striatal reactivity associated with impulsivity. *Molecular Psychiatry, 14,* 60–70.

Freimuth, M. (2005). *Hidden addictions*. Lanham, MD: Aaronson Press.

Friedmann, P. D., Hendrickson, J. C., Gerstein, D. R., & Zhang, Z. (2004). The effect of matching comprehensive services to patients' needs on drug use improvement in addiction treatment. *Addiction, 99*, 962–972.

Gamblers Anonymous International Service Office. (n.d.). *History*. Retrieved from *www.gamblersanonymous.org/history.html*.

Gilbert, P., & Leahy, R. L. (Eds.).(2007). *The therapeutic relationship in the cognitive and behavioral psychotherapies*. New York: Routledge.

Goldbeck, R., Myatt, P., & Aitchison, T. (1997). End-of-treatment self-efficacy: A predictor of abstinence. *Addiction, 92*, 313–324.

Grant, B. F., Stinson, F. S., Dawson, D. A., Chou, S. P., Dufour, M. C., Compton, W., et al. (2004). Prevalence and co-occurrence of substance use disorders and independent mood and anxiety disorders: Results from the National Epidemiologic Survey on Alcohol and Related Conditions. *Archives of General Psychiatry, 61*, 807–816.

Grant, J. E., Brewer, J. A., & Potenza, M. N. (2006). The neurobiology of substance and behavioral addictions. *CNS Spectrums, 11*, 924–930.

Grant, J. E., & Potenza, M. N. (2007). Treatments for pathological gambling and other impulse control disorders. In P. E. Nathan & J. M. Gorman (Eds.), *A guide to treatments that work* (3rd ed., pp. 561–577). New York: Oxford University Press.

Greenberger, D., & Padesky, C. A. (1995). *Mind over mood: A cognitive therapy treatment manual for clients*. New York: Guilford Press.

Hasin, D. S., Stinson, F. S., Ogburn, E., & Grant, B. F. (2007). Prevalence, correlates, disability, and comorbidity of DSM-IV alcohol abuse and dependence in the United States: Results from the National Epidemiologic Survey on Alcohol and Related Conditions. *Archives of General Psychiatry, 64*, 830–842.

Hautekeete, M., Cousin, I., & Graziani, P. (1999). Pensées dysfonctionnelles de l'alcoolo-dépendance: Un test du modèle de Beck: Schémas anticipatoires, soulageants et permissifs. *Journal de Thérapie Comportementale et Cognitive, 9*, 108–112.

Hawkins, J., Catalano, R. F., & Miller, J. Y. (1992). Risk and protective factors for alcohol and other drug problems in adolescence and early adulthood: Implications for substance abuse prevention. *Psychological Bulletin, 112*, 64–105.

Hides, L., Carroll, S., Catania, L., Cotton, S., Baker, A., Scaffidi, A., et al. (2010). Outcomes of an integrated cognitive behaviour therapy (CBT) treatment program for co-occurring depression and substance misuse in young people. *Journal of Affective Disorders, 121*, 169–174.

Higgins, S. T., Sigmon, S. C., & Heil, S. H. (2008). Drug abuse and dependence. In D. H. Barlow (Ed.), *Clinical handbook of psychological disorders: A step-by-step treatment manual* (4th ed., pp. 547–577). New York: Guilford Press.

Hudson, J. I., Hiripi, E., Pope, H. R., & Kessler, R. C. (2007). The prevalence and correlates of eating disorders in the National Comorbidity Survey Replication. *Biological Psychiatry, 61*, 348–358.

Hughes, J. R., Helzer, J. E., & Lindberg, S. A. (2006). Prevalence of DSM/ICD-defined nicotine dependence. *Drug and Alcohol Dependence, 85*, 91–102.

Hunt, W. A., Barnett, L. W., & Branch, L. G. (1971). Relapse rates in addiction programs. *Journal of Clinical Psychology, 27,* 455–456.

Irvin, J. E., Bowers, C. A., Dunn, M. E., & Wong, M. C. (1999). Efficacy of relapse prevention: A meta-analytic review. *Journal of Consulting and Clinical Psychology, 67,* 563–570.

Islam, M., Day, C. A., & Conigrave, K. M. (2010). Harm reduction healthcare: From an alternative to the mainstream platform? *International Journal of Drug Policy, 21,* 131–133.

Jones, B., Corbin, W., & Fromme, K. (2001). A review of expectancy theory and alcohol consumption. *Addiction, 96,* 57–72.

Kadden, R. M., Litt, M. D., Cooney, N., Kabela, E., & Getter, H. (2001). Prospective matching of alcoholic clients to cognitive-behavioral or interactional group therapy. *Journal of Studies on Alcohol, 62,* 359–369.

Kafka, M. P. (2007). Paraphilia-related disorders: The evaluation and treatment of nonparaphilic hypersexuality. In S. R. Leiblum (Ed.), *Principles and practice of sex therapy* (4th ed., pp. 442–476). New York: Guilford Press.

Kalichman, S. C., Cherry, C., Cain, D., Pope, H., & Kalichman, M. (2005). Psychosocial and behavioral correlates of seeking sex partners on the Internet among HIV-positive men. *Annals of Behavioral Medicine, 30,* 243–250.

Kapson, H., & Haaga, D. F. (2010). Depression vulnerability moderates the effects of cognitive behavior therapy in a randomized controlled trial for smoking cessation. *Behavior Therapy, 41,* 447–460.

Karoll, B. R. (2010). Applying social work approaches, harm reduction, and practice wisdom to better serve those with alcohol and drug disorders. *Journal of Social Work, 10,* 263–281.

Kessler, R. C., Hwang, I., Petukhova, M., Sampson, N. A., Winters, K. C., & Shaffer, H. J. (2008). DSM-IV pathological gambling in the National Comorbidity Survey Replication. *Psychological Medicine, 38,* 1351–1360.

Kobus, K., & Henry, D. B. (2010). Interplay of network position and peer substance use in early adolescent cigarette, alcohol, and marijuana use. *Journal of Early Adolescence, 30,* 225–245.

Kreek, M. J., Nielsen, D. A., Butelman, E. R., & LaForge, K. S. (2005). Genetic influences on impulsivity, risk taking, stress responsivity and vulnerability to drug abuse and addiction. *Nature Neuroscience, 8,* 1450–1457.

Ladouceur, R., Sylvain, C., Boutin, C., Lachance, S., Doucet, C., Leblond, J., & Jacques, C. (2001). Cognitive treatment of pathological gambling. *Journal of Nervous and Mental Disease, 189,* 774–780.

Ladouceur, R., & Walker, M. (1996). A cognitive perspective on gambling. In P. M. Salkovskis (Ed.), *Trends in cognitive therapy* (pp. 89–120). Oxford, UK: Wiley.

Larimer, M. E., Palmer, R. S., & Marlatt, G. A. (1999). Relapse prevention: An overview of Marlatt's cognitive-behavioral model. *Alcohol Research and Health, 23,* 151–160.

Lawrence, A. J., Luty, J., Bogdan, N. A., Sahakian, B. J., & Clark, L. (2009). Impulsivity and response inhibition in alcohol dependence and problem gambling. *Psychopharmacologia, 207,* 163–172.

Liese, B. S., & Franz, R. A. (1996). Treating substance use disorders with cognitive therapy: Lessons learned and implications for the future. In P. Salkovskis (Ed.), *Frontiers of cognitive therapy* (pp. 470–508). New York: Guilford Press.

Linehan, M. M. (1993). *Skills training manual for borderline personality disorder.* New York: Guilford Press.

Litt, M. D., Kadden, R. M., Cooney, N. L., & Kabela, E. (2003). Coping skills and treatment outcomes in cognitive-behavioral and interactional group therapy for alcoholism. *Journal of Consulting and Clinical Psychology, 71*, 118–128.

MacMaster, S. A. (2004). Harm reduction: A new perspective on substance abuse services. *Social Work, 49*, 356–363.

Malat, J., Leszcz, M., Negrete, J., Turner, N., Collins, J., Liu, E., & Toneatto, T. (2008). Interpersonal group psychotherapy for comorbid alcohol dependence and non-psychotic psychiatric disorders. *American Journal on Addictions, 17*, 402–407.

Marks, D. F., & Sykes, C. M. (2002). Randomized controlled trial of cognitive behavioural therapy for smokers living in a deprived area of London: Outcome at one-year follow-up. *Psychology, Health, and Medicine, 7*, 17–24.

Marlatt, G. A., & Donovan, D. M. (Eds.). (2005). *Relapse prevention: Maintenance strategies in the treatment of addictive behaviors* (2nd ed.). New York: Guilford Press.

Marlatt, G. A., & Witkiewitz, K. (2005). Relapse prevention for alcohol and drug problems. In G. A. Marlatt & D. M. Donovan (Eds.), *Relapse prevention: Maintenance strategies in the treatment of addictive behaviors* (2nd ed., pp. 1–44). New York: Guilford Press.

Marshal, M. P. (2003). For better or for worse? The effects of alcohol use on marital functioning. *Clinical Psychology Review, 23*, 959–997.

Maude-Griffin, P. M., Hahenstein, J. M., Humfleet, G. L., Reilly, P. M., Tusel, D. J., & Hall, S. M. (1998). Superior efficacy of cognitive behavioral therapy for urban crack cocaine abusers: Main and matching effects. *Journal of Consulting and Clinical Psychology, 66*, 832–837.

McBride, K. R., Reece, M., & Sanders, S. (2008). Using the Sexual Compulsivity Scale to predict outcomes of sexual behavior in young adults. *Sexual Addiction and Compulsivity, 15*, 97–115.

McCarty, D., Gustafson, D. H., Wisdom, J. P., Ford, J., Choi, D., Molfenter, T., et al. (2007). The Network for the Improvement of Addiction Treatment (NIATx): Enhancing access and retention. *Drug and Alcohol Dependence, 88*, 138–145.

McCrady, B. S. (2008). Alcohol use disorders. In D. H. Barlow (Ed.), *Clinical handbook of psychological disorders: A step-by-step treatment manual* (4th ed., pp. 492–546). New York: Guilford Press.

McLellan, A. T., Luborsky, L., Cacciola, J., Griffith, J., McGahan, P., & O'Brien, C. P. (1985). *Guide to the Addiction Severity Index: Background, administration, and field testing results.* Washington, DC: U.S. Government Printing Office.

Merikangas, K. R., Dierker, L. C., & Szatmari, P. (1998). Psychopathology among offspring of parents with substance abuse and/or anxiety disorders: A high-risk study. *Journal of Child Psychology & Psychiatry and Allied Disciplines, 39*, 711–720.

Miller, W. R. (1983). Controlled drinking: A history and a critical review. *Journal of Studies on Alcohol, 44*, 68–83.

Miller, W. R., Brown, J. M., Simpson, T. L., Handmaker, N. S., Bien, T. H., Luckie, L. F., et al. (1995). What works? A methodological analysis of the alcohol treatment literature. In R. K. Hester & W. R. Miller (Eds.), *Handbook of alcoholism treatment approaches: Effective alternatives* (pp. 12–44). Boston: Allyn & Bacon.

Miller, W. R., & Rollnick, S. (2002). *Motivational interviewing: Preparing people for change* (2nd ed.). New York: Guilford Press.

Miller, W. R., & Wilbourne, P. L. (2002). Mesa grande: A methodological analysis of clinical trials of treatments for alcohol use disorders. *Addiction, 97*, 265–277.

Moeller, F., Barratt, E. S., Dougherty, D. M., Schmitz, J. M., & Swann, A. C. (2001). Psychiatric aspects of impulsivity. *American Journal of Psychiatry, 158*, 1783–1793.

Moeller, F., & Dougherty, D. M. (2002). Impulsivity and substance abuse: What is the connection? *Addictive Disorders and Their Treatment, 1*, 3–10.

Moeller, F. G., Dougherty, D. M., Barratt, E. S., Schmitz, J. M., Swann, A. C., & Grabowski, J. (2001). The impact of impulsivity on cocaine use and retention in treatment. *Journal of Substance Abuse Treatment, 21*, 193–198.

Monti, P. M., Abrams, D. B., Binkoff, J. A., Zwick, W. R., Liepman, M. R., Nirenbergm T. J., et al. (1990). Communication skills training, communication skills training with family, and cognitive-behavioral mood management training for alcoholics. *Journal of Studies on Alcohol, 51*, 263–270.

Monti, P. M., Kadden, R. M., Rohsenow, D. J., Cooney, N. L., & Abrams, D. B. (2002). *Treating alcohol dependence: A coping skills training guide* (2nd ed.). New York: Guilford Press.

Monti, P. M., Rohsenow, D. J., Swift, R. M., Gulliver, S. B., Colby, S. M., Mueller, T. I., et al. (2001). Naltrexone and cue exposure with coping and communication skills training for alcoholics: Treatment process and one-year outcomes. *Alcoholism: Clinical and Experimental Research, 25*, 1634–1647.

Moos, R. (2007). Theory-based active ingredients of effective treatments for substance use disorders. *Drug and Alcohol Dependence, 88*, 109–121.

Morahan-Martin, J., & Schumacher, P. (1999). Incidence and correlates of pathological Internet use among college students. *Computers and Human Behavior, 16*, 1–17.

Morgenstern, J., & Longabaugh, R. (2000). Cognitive-behavioral treatment for alcohol dependence: A review of evidence for its hypothesized mechanisms of action. *Addiction, 95*, 1475–1490.

Morrison, N. (2001). Group cognitive therapy: Treatment of choice or sub-optimal option? *Behavioural and Cognitive Psychotherapy, 29*, 311–332.

Muench, F., Morgenstern, J., Hollander, E., Irwin, T. W., O'Leary, A., Parsons, J. T., et al. (2007). The consequences of compulsive sexual behavior: The preliminary reliability and validity of the Compulsive Sexual Behavior Consequences Scale. *Sexual Addiction and Compulsivity, 14*, 207–220.

Muñoz, R. F., Ippen, C. G., Rao, S., Le, H., & Dwyer, E. V. (2000). *Manual for group cognitive-behavioral therapy of major depression: A reality management approach.* San Francisco: University of California, San Francisco. Retrieved from *www.medschool.ucsf.edu/latino/manuals.aspx#GroupCognitiveBehavioralTherapyofMajorDepression.*

Niaura, R. S., Rohsenow, D. J., Binkoff, J., Monti, P. M., Pedraza, M., & Abrams, D. B. (1988). Relevance of cue reactivity to understanding alcohol and smoking relapse. *Journal of Abnormal Psychology, 97,* 133–152.

Norcross, J. C., Krebs, P. M., & Prochaska, J. O. (2011). Stages of change. *Journal of Clinical Psychology: In Session, 67,* 143–154.

Ockene, J., Kristeller, J. L., Goldberg, R., Ockene, I., Merriam, P., & Barrett, S. (1992). Smoking cessation and severity of disease: The Coronary Artery Smoking Intervention Study. *Health Psychology, 11,* 119–126.

Office of National Drug Control Policy. (2004). *The economic costs of drug abuse in the United States, 1992–2002.* Retrieved from *www.ncjrs.gov/ondcppubs/publications/pdf/economic_costs.pdf.*

Ojehagen, A., & Berglund, M. (1989). Changes of drinking goals in a two-year outpatient alcoholic treatment program. *Addictive Behaviors, 14,* 1–9.

Pabst, A., Baumeister, S. E., & Kraus, L. (2010). Alcohol-expectancy dimensions and alcohol consumption at different ages in the general population. *Journal of Studies on Alcohol and Drugs, 71,* 46–53.

Padesky, C. A., & Greenberger, D. (1995). *Clinician's guide to "Mind Over Mood."* New York: Guilford Press.

Palmer, R. S., Murphy, M. K., Piselli, A., & Ball, S. A. (2009). Substance user treatment dropout from client and clinician perspectives: A pilot study. *Substance Use & Misuse, 44,* 1021–1038.

Paterson, R. J. (2000). *The assertiveness workbook: How to express your ideas and stand up for yourself at work and in relationships.* Oakland, CA: New Harbinger.

Perry, J. L., & Carroll, M. E. (2008). The role of impulsive behavior in drug abuse. *Psychopharmacology, 200,* 1–26.

Polivy, J., & Herman, C. P. (2002). If at first you don't succeed: False hopes of self-change. *American Psychologist, 57,* 677–689.

Potenza, M. N., & Taylor, J. R. (2009). Found in translation: Understanding impulsivity and related constructs through integrative preclinical and clinical research. *Biological Psychiatry, 66,* 714–716.

Prochaska, J. O., & DiClemente, C. C. (1982). Transtheoretical therapy: Toward a more integrative model of change. *Psychotherapy, 19,* 276–288.

Prochaska, J. O., & DiClemente, C. C. (2005). The transtheoretical approach. In J. C. Norcross & M. R. Goldfried (Eds.), *Handbook of psychotherapy integration* (2nd ed., pp. 147–171). New York: Oxford University Press.

Project MATCH Research Group. (1997). Matching alcoholism treatments to client heterogeneity: Project MATCH posttreatment drinking outcomes. *Journal of Studies on Alcohol, 58,* 7–29.

Reilly, P. M., Shopshire, M. S., Durazzo, T. C., & Campbell, T. A. (2002). *Anger management for substance abuse and mental health clients: Participant workbook* (DHHS Publication No. SMA 02-3662). Retrieved from *www.kap.samhsa.gov/products/manuals/pdfs/anger2.pdf.*

Roberts, L. J., & Marlatt, G. A. (1999). Harm reduction. In P. J. Ott, R. E. Tarter,

& R. T. Ammerman (Eds.), *Sourcebook on substance abuse: Etiology, epidemiology, assessment, and treatment* (pp. 389–398). Boston: Allyn & Bacon.

Robinson, T. E., & Berridge, K. C. (1993). The neural basis of drug craving: An incentive-sensitization theory of addiction. *Brain Research Review, 8,* 247–291.

Rohsenow, D. J., Monti, P. M., Rubonis, A. V., Gulliver, S. B., Colby, S M., Binkoff, J. A., et al. (2001). Cue exposure with coping skills training and communication skills training for alcohol dependence: Six and twelve month outcomes. *Addiction, 96,* 1161–1174.

Rosen, C. S. (2000). Is the sequencing of change processes by stage consistent across health problems? A meta-analysis. *Health Psychology, 19,* 593–604.

Rotgers, F., & Nguyen, T. A. (2006). Substance abuse. In P. J. Bieling, R. E. McCabe, & M. M. Antony, *Cognitive-behavioral therapy in groups* (pp. 298–323). New York: Guilford Press.

Safran, J. D., & Segal, Z. V. (1990). *Interpersonal process in cognitive therapy.* New York: Basic Books.

Sanchez-Craig, M., & Lei, H. (1986). Disadvantages of imposing the goal of abstinence on problem drinkers: An empirical study. *British Journal of Addictions, 81,* 505–512.

Sarnecki, J., Traynor, R., & Clune, M. (2008). Cue fascination: A new vulnerability in drug addiction. *Behavioral and Brain Sciences, 31,* 458–459.

Shaffer, H. J., Hall, M. N., & Vander Bilt, J. (1999). Estimating the prevalence of disordered gambling behavior in the United States and Canada: A research synthesis. *American Journal of Public Health, 89,* 1369–1376.

Shaffer, H. J., & LaPlante, D. A. (2005). The treatment of gambling related disorders. In G. A. Marlatt & D. M. Donovan (Eds.), *Relapse prevention: Maintenance strategies in the treatment of addictive behaviors* (2nd ed., pp. 276–332). New York: Guilford Press.

Shiffman, S., Hickcox, M., Paty, J. A., Gnys, M., Kassel, J. D., & Richards, T. J. (1996). Progression from a smoking lapse to relapse: Prediction from abstinence violation effects, nicotine dependence, and lapse characteristics. *Journal of Consulting and Clinical Psychology, 64,* 993–1002.

Shiffman, S., Paty, J. A., Gnys, M., Kassel, J. D., & Hickcox, M. (1996). First lapses to smoking: Within subjects analysis of real time reports. *Journal of Consulting and Clinical Psychology, 64,* 366–379.

Sobell, L. C., & Sobell, M. B. (2011). *Group therapy for substance use disorders: A motivational cognitive-behavioral approach.* New York: Guilford Press.

Sobell, L. C., Sobell, M. B., & Agrawal, S. (2009). Randomized controlled trial of a cognitive-behavioral motivational intervention in a group versus individual format for substance use disorders. *Psychology of Addictive Behaviors, 23,* 672–683.

Sobell, M. B., & Sobell, L. C. (1993). *Problem drinkers: Guided self-change treatment.* New York: Guilford Press.

Stinson, F. S., Grant, B. F., Dawson, D. A., Ruan, W. J., Juang, B., & Saha, T. (2005). Comorbidity between DSM-IV alcohol and specific drug use disorders in the United States: Results from the national Epidemiologic Survey on Alcohol and Related Conditions. *Drug and Alcohol Dependence, 80,* 105–116.

Striegel-Moore, R. H., & Franko, D. L. (2008). Should binge eating disorder be included in the DSM-V?: A critical review of the state of the evidence. *Annual Review of Clinical Psychology, 4*, 305–324.

Substance Abuse and Mental Health Services Administration. (2011). *Results from the 2010 National Survey on Drug Use and Health: Summary of national findings* (NSDUH Series H-41, HHS Publication No. SMA 11-4658). Rockville, MD: Author. Retrieved from *www.samhsa.gov/data/NSDUH.aspx.*

Substance Abuse and Mental Health Services Administration, Center for Behavioral Health Statistics and Quality. (2010, December 28). *The DAWN Report: Highlights of the 2009 Drug Abuse Warning Network (DAWN) findings on drug-related emergency department visits.* Rockville, MD: Author. Retrieved from *www.oas.samhsa.gov/2k10/DAWN034/EDHighlightsHTML.pdf.*

Swendsen, J., Conway, K. P., Degenhardt, L., Glantz, M., Jin, R., Merikangas, K. R., et al. (2010). Mental disorders as risk factors for substance use, abuse and dependence: Results from the 10-year follow-up of the National Comorbidity Survey. *Addiction, 105*, 1117–1128.

Sylvain, C., Ladouceur, R., & Boisvert, J. M. (1997). Cognitive and behavioral treatment of pathological gambling: A controlled study. *Journal of Consulting and Clinical Psychology, 65*, 727–732.

Tison P., & Hautekeete M. (1998). Mise en évidence de schémas cognitifs dysfonctionnels chez des toxicomanes. *Journal de Thérapie Comportementale et Cognitive, 2*, 43–49.

Tzilos, G. K., Rhodes, G. L., Ledgerwood, D. M., & Greenwald, M. K. (2009). Predicting cocaine group treatment outcome in cocaine-abusing methadone patients. *Experimental and Clinical Psychopharmacology, 17*, 320–325.

Urbán, R., & Demetrovics, Z. (2010). Smoking outcome expectancies: A multiple indicator and multiple cause (MIMIC) model. *Addictive Behaviors, 35*, 632–635.

Velasquez, M. M., Maurer, G. G., Crouch, C., & DiClemente, C. C. (2001). *Group treatment for substance abuse.* New York: Guilford Press.

Weinberg, M. S., Williams, C. J., Kleiner, S., & Irizarry, Y. (2010). Pornography, normalization, and empowerment. *Archives of Sexual Behavior, 39*, 1389–1401.

Wenzel, A., Brown, G. K., & Beck, A. T. (2009). *Cognitive therapy for suicidal patients: Scientific and clinical applications.* Washington, DC: APA Books.

Wenzel, A., Brown, G. K., & Karlin, B. E. (2011). *Cognitive behavioral therapy for depressed veterans and military servicemembers: Therapist manual.* Washington, DC: U.S. Department of Veterans Affairs.

Wheeler, J. G., George, W. H., & Stoner, S. A. (2005). Enhancing the relapse prevention model for sex offenders: Adding recidivism risk reduction therapy to target offenders' dynamic risk needs. In G. A. Marlatt & D. M. Donovan (Eds.), *Relapse prevention: Maintenance strategies in the treatment of addictive behaviors* (2nd ed., pp. 333–362). New York: Guilford Press.

White, J. R. (2000). Depression. In J. R. White & A. S. Freeman (Eds.), *Cognitive-behavioral group therapy for specific problems and populations* (pp. 29–61). Washington, DC: APA Books.

Whiteside, S. P., & Lynam, D. R. (2001). The five factor model and impulsivity:

Using a structural model of personality to understand impulsivity. *Personality and Individual Differences, 30,* 669–689.

Wilfley, D. E., Wilson, G. T., & Agras, W. S. (2003). The clinical significance of binge eating disorder. *International Journal of Eating Disorders, 34*(Suppl.), S96–S106.

Witkiewitz, K., & Marlatt, G. A. (2004). Relapse prevention for alcohol and drug problems: That was Zen, this is Tao. *American Psychologist, 59,* 224–235.

Woody, G. E., Luborsky, L., McLellan, A. T., & O'Brien, C. P. (1990). Corrections and revised analyses for psychotherapy in methadone maintenance programs. *Archives of General Psychiatry, 47,* 788–789.

World Health Organization. (2010). *Global strategy to reduce the harmful use of alcohol.* Geneva, Switzerland: Author. Retrieved from *www.who.int/substance_abuse/msbalcstragegy.pdf.*

World Health Organization. (2011). *Tobacco Free Initiative (TFI): Why tobacco is a public health priority.* Retrieved from *www.who.int/tobacco/health_priority/en.*

Xie, H., McHugo, G. J., Fox, M. B., & Drake, R. E. (2005). Special section on relapse prevention: Substance abuse relapse in a ten-year prospective follow-up of clients with mental and substance use disorders. *Psychiatric Services, 56,* 1282–1287.

Yalom, I., & Leszcz, M. (2005). *The theory and practice of group psychotherapy* (5th ed.). New York: Basic Books.

Young, K. (2007). Cognitive behavior therapy with Internet addicts: Treatment outcomes and implications. *CyberPsychology and Behavior, 10,* 671–679.

Young, K. S. (1998). Internet addiction: The emergence of a new clinical disorder. *CyberPsychology and Behavior, 1,* 237–244.

Young, K. S. (2008). Internet sex addiction: Risk factors, stages of development, and treatment. *American Behavioral Scientist, 52,* 21–37.

Index